"Outstanding"

"St. John's wort may be the best natural remedy since chicken soup for improving your outlook on life, and gives new hope to millions. This book provides outstanding, practical information in a warm and friendly style, and reflects the healing quality of Dr. Cass' years of work as a holistic psychiatrist."

Jack Canfield
Co-author: "Chicken Soup for the Soul"

"Easy-to-Read"

"A clear, concise easy-to-read book. I would recommend it for everyone's library."

Earl Mindell, R.Ph., Ph.D.
Author: "Earl Mindell's Supplement Bible,"
"Earl Mindell's Herb Bible," and
"Earl Mindell's Anti-aging Bible"

"Practical"

"Finally, a practical book on St John's wort. Dr. Cass has done a great job. I used it immediately to help a patient switch from a drug to this natural alternative."

Dharma Singh Khalsa, M.D.
Author: "Brain Longevity" and "The Pain Cure"
President/Medical Director Alzheimer's Prevention
Foundation, Tucson, Az.

"Inspiring and Remarkable"

"Dr. Cass had done an inspiring and remarkable synthesis on the natural treatment of the disease of our century. Her commitment to health and healing is most apparent in this book, which I highly recommend to physicians and general public alike."

Carlos Warter, M.D., Ph.D.
Author: "Who Do You Think You Are?"
President World Health Foundation
for Development & Peace

"Terrific"

"Now Dr. Hyla Cass, a psychiatrist who utilizes a broad range of therapies, shares her knowledge and perspective regarding the proper role of this marvelous herb. This is a terrific book that anybody who is concerned about depression should get right away."

Melvyn R. Werbach, M.D.
Author: "Nutritional Influences on Illness"

"Holistic"

"Dr. Hyla Cass tells us how and why [St. John's wort] works, and when it might be helpful. Even more important, she shows us how we can use it as part of an individualized and holistic approach for those of us who suffer from depression."

James S. Gordon, M.D.
Author: "Manifesto For A New Medicine,"
Clinical Professor of Psychiatry, Georgetown University
School of Medicine, Director and Founder,
Center for Mind-Body Medicine

ST. JOHN'S
WORT

Nature's Blues Buster

HYLA CASS, MD

Avery Publishing Group
Garden City Park, New York

The therapeutic procedures in this book are based on the training, personal experiences, and research of the author. Because each person and situation are unique, the author and publisher urge the reader to check with a qualified health professional before using any procedure where there is any question to appropriateness.

The publisher does not advocate the use of any particular health program, but believes the information presented in this book should be available to the public.

Because there is always some risk involved, the author and publisher are not responsible for any adverse effects or consequences resulting from the use of any of the suggestions, preparations, or procedures described in this book. Please do not use the book if you are unwilling to assume the risk. Feel free to consult with a physician or other qualified health professional. It is a sign of wisdom, not cowardice, to seek a second or third opinion.

Cover design: Tim Boylan
Typesetters: Al Berotti and
   Elaine V. McCaw
In-house editor: Lisa James

Avery Publishing Group, Inc.
120 Old Broadway
Garden City Park, New York 11040
1-800-548-5757

Publisher's Cataloging-in-Publication

Cass, Hyla.
    St. John's Wort : nature's blues buster / by Hyla Cass. — 1st
ed.
      p. cm.
      Includes bibliographical references and index.
      ISBN: 0-89529-834-1

      1. Depression, Mental—Alternative treatment. 2. Hypericum
perforatum—Therapeutic use.   I. Title.

RC537.C37 1998   616.85'27061
                          QBI97-41308

Printed in the United States of America

10   9   8

Contents

To the blessed memory of my father,
Dr. Isadore Morris Cass,
who taught me healing

Acknowledgments

I stand on the shoulders of the ancients, whose knowledge of nature's medicine survives, thanks to all those who have carried on the tradition, sometimes at great risk. The current resurgence of interest holds great hope for the future. As we recognize and utilize these gifts of Mother Earth, let us thank her accordingly.

I thank all my teachers for their information and inspiration over many years and in many diverse areas. Among my greatest teachers I include my patients, who have not only challenged me to look beyond the ordinary for their healing, but have encouraged me in other countless ways.

I offer special thanks to Joerg Gruenwald, Ph.D., my European Scientific Research Consultant, for generously sharing his knowledge and experience, and to Müggenburg Extrakt-North America, for making their private research portfolio available to me.

I want to thank many who shared with me their information and support, including: Mark Blumenthal, Peggy and Bill Brevoort, Dan Bielen, Don Brown, Jerry Cott, Floyd Leaders, Rob McCaleb, Michael McGuffin, Ed Smith, Roy Upton, and Terry Willard.

I am immensely grateful to the members of my alternative medicine support group, who have taught me much of what I know. They continue to educate and inspire me and each other, and are also my dear friends: Drs. Moses Albalas, David Allen, John Finnegan, Joe D. Goldstrich, Allen Green, Hans Gruen, Jesse Hanley, Uzzi Reiss, Michael Rosenbaum, Priscilla Slagle, Murray Susser, Cynthia Watson, Mel Werbach, and Janet Zand.

I thank my friends who have inspired, advised and, above all, believed in me: Jim Autry, Arline and Harold Brecher, Joel Edelman, Marilyn Ferguson ("write your passion"), Dori Glover, Bill Kastenberg, Jack Klein, Lyn and Norman Lear, Tim Piering, Penny Price, Jim Strohecker (my "manager"), Carlos Warter, and Andrew Weil.

I owe a heartfelt debt to my loving family: my mother, Miriam Cass, who has always believed in me; my daughter, Alison, who is ever helpful—and knows when not to interrupt my writing; and my sisters, Sharon Toole, Judy Finkelstein, and Elaine Cass, who are there for listening, feedback, and encouragement.

I thankfully acknowledge my publisher, Rudy Shur, a true *mensch*, who challenged me to write this book, and patiently and generously guided me throughout; Dave Tuttle, who helped compile information; and Lisa James, my editor, who, with utmost patience and professionalism, helped shape the book, and hurried me along when needed.

Above all, I want to thank Terrence McNally, whose love, humor, patience, and support allowed me to complete this enormous task in one piece, and whose editorial input made an enormous contribution to the book.

Preface

St. John's wort, an old herbal remedy and common plant, is rapidly becoming the most talked-about new treatment for depression here in North America. From *Newsweek* and *Time* to major television shows, we are hearing of this natural treatment—as good as conventional antidepressants, without the side effects, and at a fraction the cost. Sales have skyrocketed: A European company that shipped 1 ton in all of 1996 shipped 5 tons in the month following the start of major-media publicity. Obviously, people are looking for alternatives, and may have found it here. Many are now wondering how to view this information: Is it as good as it sounds, or is it the flavor or the month, soon to be found ineffective, or worse?

We are all bombarded daily with confusing, conflicting health news. In the last few years, we have seen the introduction of many novel products such as DHEA and melatonin, along with a bewildering assortment of amino acids and even more exotic nutrients. Be it a vitamin, mineral, herb, or hormone, something new seems to burst onto the scene almost daily, with experts calling it the "ultimate answer." The next month, however, *other* experts tell us that this new "miracle substance" isn't all it's cracked up to be, or even dangerous. Even the familiar vitamins A, C, and E get their share of good and bad press. It is confusing to know whom to believe. We want to know if these products really work. Are they safe? Could there be as-yet undiscovered negative effects to be revealed only after long-term use?

This supplement revolution is part of growing shift in our concepts and practice of health care. While costs continue to rise and problems mount in the delivery system, technologically based modern medicine has failed to keep its promise of a cure for every ill. By the millions, people are looking for other, more natural choices. A landmark study by Harvard University's Dr. David Eisenberg, published in the respected *New England Journal of Medicine,* reported that 34 percent of the American health dollar was being spent on some form of alternative therapy. That was in 1994, and the figures have risen significantly since then.

The pharmaceutical industry, like the rest of modern medicine, has not fulfilled its promise. Drugs designed to cure or alleviate illness often have serious side effects, some worse than the condition they are meant to treat. Hundreds of people even die each year from the toxic effects of these prescribed medications! On the other hand, when used as recommended, herbs produce few side effects, and an overdose of most herbs is unlikely to have serious consequences. Herbs have a long and successful track record, providing health benefits to countless generations of people across many lands and cultures. It is only in the United States, where science and technology so firmly rule, that the herbal traditions have been all but lost.

As we've seen, there is an overwhelming demand from the public for more natural substances, plus major media attention focused on herbs in general and St. John's wort in particular. Specific questions arise: What is St. John's wort? Does it work? How does it work? How does it compare with conventional drug treatments? Is it for me, or someone I care about who is suffering from depression? How long does it take to work? If I am already on an antidepressant, should I switch? How do I do that? How long can I stay on it? Are there side effects? What are the long-term effects?

After hearing these questions over and over, I decided to draw upon my own knowledge of the use of St. John's wort for depression, review the available research information, and provide a simple guide to its use. I also wanted to describe how this herb can be successfully combined with the other natural products that I have found over many years of clinical practice to address the underlying cause of a disorder, rather than just treating the symptoms.

Depression is a significant problem in today's world, and its incidence is increasing exponentially. It reflects imbalance not only within the individual, but also within our society and environment. Our bodies are out of balance on a biochemical level. We do not have the proper basic ingredients for good mental and physical health. Contributing factors are toxic air, food, and water, plus poor diet and inadequate food sources that are manufactured or grown for convenience and profit rather than for proper nutritional value. The depression that results from these factors is then commonly treated with prescription drugs with many unwanted side effects. Now we have a natural herb that has received massive exposure for its many benefits in overcoming depression. While many see it as new wonder, it has been used for centuries. Moreover, for the past five years it has been the treatment of choice in Europe, outnumbering all antidepressant prescriptions.

I have written this book to help you, the reader, take charge of your own emotional well-being. My goal is to educate you about possible choices available in this rapidly expanding and often confusing new world of alternative medicine. I have drawn from real-life situations in my practice of psychiatry and complementary medicine to give you a first-hand look at both the problems and the solutions.

Hyla Cass, M.D.
Los Angeles, California

St. John's wort doth charm all witches away,
If gathered at midnight on the saint's holy day.
Any devils and witches have no power to harm
Those that gather the plant for a charm.
Rub the lintels with that red juicy flower;
No thunder nor tempest will then have the power
To hurt or hinder your house; and bind
Round your neck a charm of a similar kind.

poem dating from about A.D. 1400

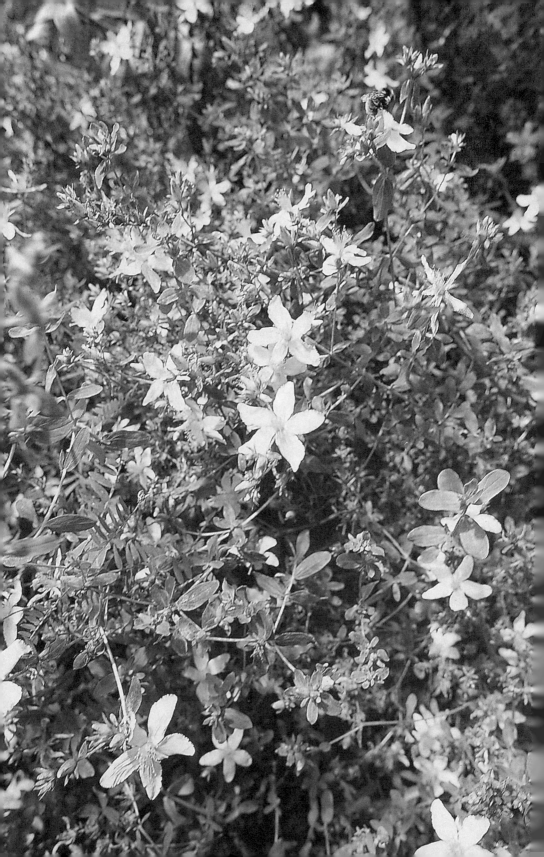

Introduction

Depression wears many faces. Sometimes it is a melancholy feeling. Sometimes, it is fatigue, apathy, or anxiety. There are even times when it is several of these things at once. But it always feels like it's holding you back from enjoying life the way you should. Now, there's a solution that does not involve synthetic drugs and their side effects. It is an herb called St. John's wort.

Throughout my many years as a practicing psychiatrist, I have searched for natural remedies to help my clients. I am well aware of the benefits of conventional drugs, and have employed them in my practice when appropriate. But I am also aware of the side effects and expense associated with synthetic antidepressants such as Prozac. There are many people—perhaps millions—who will do as well, often better, on St. John's wort.

I have used St. John's wort extensively, and can testify that it is as effective as it is gentle. I have seen this remarkable herb help bring welcome relief to many of my clients. People who had known depression all their lives have been overjoyed to find a new sense of peace and calm. Freed from sadness and anxiety, they have gained new insight into their problems and concerns, and have been able to tackle these issues—often for the first time in years. As a therapist, I have found this experience to be deeply gratifying.

Excited by the benefits of St. John's wort and similar remedies, I have read extensively in the field, exchanged opinions and information with my colleagues, and contributed to many articles and books on the subject. While this remarkable herb has not yet been widely studied in this country, research done around the world has testified to its powers. What doctors have found is that St. John's wort is not only useful in treating certain types of depression, including seasonal affective disorder, but that it has infection-fighting and immunity-enhancing effects that make it a promising treatment for disorders ranging from skin infections to AIDS. It also seems to be especially helpful for women in its ability to fight premenstrual syndrome, menstrual cramps, and the symptoms associated with menopause.

Of course, no medicine, natural or synthetic, is a cure-all, and St. John's wort is no exception. At this time, it is not recommended as a sole treatment for major depression, nor is it recommended for bipolar disorder (also known as manic-depressive illness). In addition, there are conditions, such as chronic fatigue syndrome, that can mimic depression, and that require a comprehensive treatment program if they are to be successfully treated.

Actually, all medicines, including St. John's wort, work best when used as part of an overall treatment program. Such a program complements the use of St. John's wort with important nutrients and other herbs, as well as with a healthful diet and exercise regimen. It also takes into account the psychological factors of depression, and provides the appropriate therapy.

In this book, I explain what depression is, and how both the mind and the body affect mental health. I then tell you about the many possible benefits that St. John's wort can offer and provide information on its use, including its combination with other herbs. I not only review the studies that have been done on this plant, but provide facts on the synthetic antidepressants as well. I discuss St. John's wort's nutritional cofactors, including amino acids, vitamins, and minerals. Finally, I make lifestyle recommendations concerning diet, exercise, and stress reduction, without which no mental health program can be entirely effective.

If you suffer from depression, or if you know someone who does, I strongly urge you to learn about St. John's wort. It could make a very real difference in your life.

1

One Powerful Herb

I can't believe it! I feel normal for the first time in a long, long time—maybe ever.

Cindy, a 35-year-old working mother

Can a natural and inexpensive supplement actually relieve depression? Yes, it can. For thousands of years, people have enjoyed the health benefits of a wide variety of plants. Garlic, ginger, and willow bark are just a few of the natural remedies that have been used by people all around the world in an effort to fight off illness and preserve health. Like our ancestors, we too can find remedies within our natural surroundings. Herbs offer solutions to some of modern society's most pressing problems, including stress and depression.

One such powerful herb is St. John's wort ("wort" is Old English for plant). Known botanically by its Latin name, *Hypericum perforatum,* for its seemingly perforated leaves. Its common name comes from the fact that it blooms around June 24, the Feast of St. John. It is native to many parts of the world, including the United

States. The ancient Greeks utilized this herb for everything from the healing of wounds to the treatment of melancholy. St. John's wort is one of many herbs used by natural or wholistic physicians for years as a prime example of the healing power of nature.

In this chapter, I'll first discuss the benefits and uses of St. John's wort as a part of a natural approach to psychiatry, followed by an overview of depression and its various treatments.

THE BENEFITS OF ST. JOHN'S WORT

Contemporary herbalists have focused most of their attention on St. John's wort's ability to alleviate depression. For a fraction of the cost, this herb can be as effective as the prescription antidepressants and without the numerous side effects that often accompany these drugs. Dozens of clinical studies have demonstrated St. John's wort's remarkable ability to alleviate mild to moderate depression, as well as seasonal affective disorder (SAD), which is depression brought on by the absence of sunlight. In Germany, where much of this research has taken place, prescriptions for St. John's wort now outnumber those for Prozac (fluoxetine hydrochloride) by a ratio of at least 4 to 1, and possibly greater than that. As word has spread across the Atlantic, millions of Americans are switching from drugs such as Prozac and Zoloft (sertraline hydrochloride) to St. John's wort.

This powerful herb has a number of other medical uses, too. It can help the body fight off disease through its strong antiviral and antibacterial properties. Scientists have also confirmed the herb's value for such historical uses as wound healing, insomnia relief, and even treatment of premenstrual syndrome (PMS) and menstrual cramps (see Chapter 4).

MAKING THE NATURAL CHOICE

Sometimes, choosing a natural therapy such as St. John's wort means going against a doctor's advice, as Nancy did.

It was 9 P.M., and I was still working at my computer when the phone rang. I was surprised to hear my childhood friend, Nancy—who generally calls only to announce births, deaths, and engagements—at the other end of the line. Her urgent tone concerned me. "What do you think about St. John's wort?" she blurted out. "I know you use herbal medicines in your practice, and I have a professional question to ask you about my dad. He's been getting more and more depressed of late, so I took him to see his doctor, who recommended an antidepressant—on top of Dad's heart and blood pressure medications. I wasn't comfortable with this approach."

Earlier that week, a friend had told Nancy about St. John's wort and depression. She was intrigued by this natural alternative to antidepressant drugs and wanted to know more. Asked about his opinion of this herb, her father's doctor said that he'd never heard of it, then laughed off her question with comments about quackery, gullibility, and snake oil. Still worried about her father and unwilling to blindly follow the doctor's prescription, she went home and dialed my number. From somewhere firmly in the middle of the medical mainstream, Nancy was reaching out for help.

I told her how perfect it was that she had called. I have incorporated the use of natural substances into my psychiatric practice, reading available literature and mutually sharing information with my colleagues to keep up with the growing field. Nancy seemed relieved that she had finally found somewhere to turn.

Her questions tumbled out: "Does it really work? What do you think his doctor will say? Is it safe for him to take it with his other medications?"

She was asking all the right questions. I told her that St. John's wort would likely help her dad, but his medications were still an issue. Not a straightforward case, his use of St. John's wort would require close medical supervision by a knowledgeable doctor.

For many years I have practiced *wholistic psychiatry*, an approach that treats the mind, body, and spirit as an indivisible whole. One aspect of this approach is referred to as *orthomolecular psychiatry*, which uses natural substances rather than pharmaceutically manufactured products whenever possible. The term *orthomolecular*, coined by Nobel Prize-winning scientist Linus Pauling, means "the right molecule in the right place," and orthomolecular psychiatry relies on the use of molecules that occur naturally in the human body. I am familiar with the array of medications available, and even prescribe them at times. However, I have found the natural approach far more effective because, rather than just treating symptoms, it addresses the root cause of illness. This approach is less invasive and has longer-lasting results. We are a part of nature, so it makes perfect sense that natural products are more compatible with our biochemistry and therefore less likely to cause harm. Nature's pharmacy has become a mainstay of my practice. Disease reflects an imbalance at some level, and I often turn to herbs to help restore inner balance. For more information on the nutritional approach to psychiatry, see Chapter 8.

DEPRESSION—A VERY COMMON PROBLEM

It has been estimated that at any one time, there are 18 million Americans suffering from depression. Clinical depression is not the brief fluctuation in mood that comes from a bad day at the office or a fight with one's spouse. Rather, it is an ongoing medical illness that can consume the lives of those who are afflicted with it. Abraham Lincoln, one of many prominent people who have suffered from depression, wrote, "If what I feel were equally distributed to the whole human family, there would not be one cheerful face on earth."

For most of us, depression is a transitory feeling that passes in time, part of the ups and downs that accompany all of our lives. Clinically depressed people, on the other hand, often feel fatigued, drained of energy, empty, and hopeless. They may lose interest in the things that normally provide pleasure, even sexual activity. They may isolate themselves socially and feel quite alone. However, with proper diagnosis and treatment, including the correct use of St. John's wort where indicated, depression can often be alleviated.

There are actually several different types of depression, which we will look at more closely in Chapter 2. No individual fits any one category exactly, since depression is as variable as the persons who have it. These classifications do serve, however, as a convenient shorthand, describing symptoms, prognosis, and treatments.

Those of us who practice natural medicine have found that depression can be treated with appropriate nutritional supplements and, in many cases, with no medication at all. In the absence of treatment, on the other hand, clinically depressed individuals can become immersed in a self-perpetuating negative spiral. Let's look at both the conventional approach to depression and an approach that emphasizes the use of St. John's wort.

Standard Medical Treatments

The mainstays of traditional psychiatric treatment have

been *psychotherapy* and *medication*. Beginning with the psychological approach, to people who have experienced depression for their entire lives, "reality" feels depressing. Their mistaken beliefs and resulting behaviors tend only to reinforce their misperceptions. The goal of psychotherapy is to help patients come to terms with the world around them. It helps them to break dysfunctional patterns, and eventually to see things in a more positive light in order to achieve happier and more productive lives. More than simply a form of re-educating the patient, psychotherapy also involves "re-parenting" the patient, with the therapist providing a safe and nurturing context in which the patient can grow as an individual.

While psychotherapy was once the traditional domain of psychiatrists, times have changed. The availability of many well-trained nonmedical psychotherapists, combined with the economic realities of reductions in insurance reimbursement and the higher fees of psychiatrists as compared with those of psychotherapists, often dictates a split in patient care. Therapists, including psychologists, marriage and family counselors, and social workers, are trained to know when a problem is beyond their field of expertise, and will refer the patient for psychiatric consultation when appropriate. Thus, psychiatrists often treat only the more seriously ill individuals, or act as medication consultants rather than as primary therapists. In many of these cases, psychiatrists treat depression with antidepressant medications in an attempt to counteract the chemical imbalances in the brain. We will look at the biochemical causes of depression in Chapter 3.

Over years of laboratory research, the existing antidepressant drugs have been developed to have a very specific effect. Some of them have been in use since the 1950s, and drug therapy remains a useful tool in the treatment of psychiatric illness. We will explore the characteristics of these medications in Chapter 7.

However, the antidepressants have their drawbacks. While they may be effective 60 to 80 percent of the time in treating depression, they can exact a stiff price. Many patients stop taking them because of side effects. Common side effects of Prozac include nausea, headaches, anxiety, insomnia, drowsiness, diarrhea, dry mouth, loss of appetite, sweating, tremors, short-term memory loss, and rashes. As if all of this weren't bad enough, most antidepressants also reduce your sex drive. Studies that looked specifically at sexual dysfunction found that 30 to 40 percent of all men and women taking antidepressants suffered a drop in libido.

So what is the solution? Many effective answers to depression can be found in readily available natural substances.

St. John's Wort to the Rescue

Some of the most potent therapeutic agents are herbs (see Chapter 5). Actually concentrated foods, herbs supply our bodies with essential nourishment not found in our usual diets. They promote balance by supporting the body's basic functions, helping it to regulate and heal itself. Unlike the sledgehammer approach taken by many modern drugs, herbs work to fine-tune the body into the precision instrument that it can be.

In the treatment of various types of depression, one herb stands above all the rest: St. John's wort. I have had many opportunities to see the effects of this remarkable plant. Cindy is a good example.

A 35-year-old secretary and mother of two, Cindy had been depressed on and off for years, her intermittent attempts at psychotherapy providing only temporary relief. Her family doctor, surmising correctly that there might be a biochemical component to her depression, referred her to a psychiatrist, who prescribed Prozac.

Despite some misgivings about being dependent on a drug, Cindy accepted the recommendation out of desperation. After a few weeks, the medication began to work. Her energy level increased, and she felt better about life and herself for the first time in years. She experienced renewed interest in her husband and children. Even her job, which she had come to resent, became more enjoyable, more of a positive challenge than a burden. However, after another couple of weeks, she began to notice some troubling symptoms.

During her deepest depression, Cindy had lost all interest in sex. As she began to feel better, she expected her libido to increase as well. Instead, it declined even more. Even when she did have sex, she was unable to reach an orgasm. Both sexual problems are common side effects of Prozac and drugs of that type. In addition, she felt irritable and had trouble both falling and staying asleep. Despite her exhaustion and need for sleep, she began to dread bedtime, for more reasons than one. It didn't seem fair that she was paying so high a price for her positive change in mood!

Cindy felt betrayed, angry at herself and the world in general. While her husband, Phil, had been very supportive during her days of darkness, he was now losing his patience. He took her lack of sexual interest personally, not understanding that it wasn't her fault. She stopped taking Prozac to see if that would help, but after a few weeks, the depression began to return. Cindy's doctor offered to prescribe a different medication, but she was afraid that she would just have other problems. Fortunately, a sympathetic coworker, Joan, noticed Cindy's mood swings. Joan told Cindy about her own success with a more natural approach to psychiatry.

Cindy sat across from me relating her story. Though she was an attractive, well-dressed woman, with stylishly cut black hair and large brown eyes, there was something missing. The lack of shine in her downcast eyes, the drooping corners of her mouth, and her discouraged tone gave her away. "Doctor, I've had it. My psychiatrist wanted me to try another drug, but I just can't go through that again."

Cindy's initially promising response to Prozac confirmed that her brain chemistry was indeed out of balance. She had stopped taking Prozac six weeks earlier. But instead of giving her a synthetic chemical, I prescribed St. John's wort. I told her to take three 300-milligram capsules of the dried herb daily. A little doubtful, she asked, "How can an herb that's available without a prescription be as strong as a drug and not have side effects, either?" I explained that unlike drugs, which harshly manipulate the body's chemistry, St. John's wort works with the body to gently improve mood. Somewhat reassured, she looked up at me with a hint of her former spirit. "I know you helped Joan, so I'm willing to give it a try."

I saw Cindy four weeks later, and she was looking much better. There was now a sparkle in her eyes, and she looked directly at me instead of at the floor. "I can't believe it! I feel normal for the first time in a long, long time—maybe ever. After two weeks, I felt like I did during the early stages of Prozac, but with none of the side effects. I can think more clearly now, too. My relationship with my husband is improving daily, and," she added with a smile, "nightly, as well."

Cindy continued to take St. John's wort, reached

*a plateau of positive feeling and functioning, and got
on with her life. She comes to see me periodically
and, after more than a year, continues to do well. Her
depression is behind her. We have discussed the possibility of decreasing the dose or even discontinuing
it, but for now, she would rather let this herbal extract brighten her life than take a chance on having
a relapse.*

After years of popularity in Europe, St. John's wort
has now been recognized in the United States as a valuable tool for treating depression. Inexpensive and available without a prescription, it offers new hope to
millions of people. (We will look in detail at how you
can use St. John's wort in Chapter 5.)

Dozens of clinical studies have been conducted on St.
John's wort (see Chapter 6). More than 5,000 patients
have taken part in these investigations, including more
than 2,000 in controlled, double-blind studies—experiments in which neither the subject nor the researcher
knows who is receiving the actual substance being
tested. Time and again, the studies have shown that an
average of 70 percent of depressed patients have a significant decrease in symptoms and an increase in feelings of well-being when treated with St. John's wort.
This is the same average success rate achieved with the
prescription antidepressants, but without the side effects.

The scientific evidence has led to the widespread use
of St. John's wort in Germany, where it now accounts
for half of all the prescriptions written for depression.
Prozac, on the other hand, has only 2 percent of the
German market.

St. John's wort's powers are derived from a number
of active ingredients. Although initially considered the
main active ingredient, current research indicates that
the chemical *hypericin* does not provide the major anti-

depressant activity of St. John's wort. The hypericin content, however, is used as a convenient reference point when creating standardized extracts. For more information on hypericin and standardized extracts, see Chapter 5.

Bear in mind that depression can be a serious illness that requires medical attention. If you are frequently depressed, you should talk to your family physician or consult a psychiatrist about possible treatment options. This is true even if you are able to function normally at home or at work. You don't have to be bedridden or seriously depressed to need medical help. The secret to successfully treating depression is to uncover and treat both the biochemical *and* psychological factors that may be keeping you out of balance, so that your natural energy, initiative, and joy can shine forth. We will look at lifestyle and depression in Chapter 9.

St. John's wort is rapidly becoming the most frequently used antidepressant medication in the world. This safe and effective herb is taken by millions of Germans on a daily basis, and it is recommended by psychiatrists throughout Europe. Now, Americans have awakened to its enormous potential.

Knowledge is vital to establishing control and positive direction in your life. In the following pages, you'll learn about the various psychological, nutritional, and medical factors that are involved in treating depression, and the role of St. John's wort in such treatment. You will receive detailed information on the proper dosages to take, and you will find out about the studies that have confirmed the herb's effectiveness around the world. You'll also see how St. John's wort fares when compared with the prescription antidepressants.

2

Understanding Depression

Tears, idle tears, I know not what they mean,
Tears from the depth of some divine despair.

Alfred, Lord Tennyson

Before we look at how St. John's wort can alleviate depression, it is important to understand what we mean by the word "depression." There are potential causes of sadness in everyone's life, but most people manage to cope with their problems without becoming incapacitated. For example, you could have lost a job and felt bad for a few weeks. However, if you were unable to face the world, were in tears all the time, and were feeling like a failure, you would be suffering from a clinical depression. In other words, the feeling you were experiencing would be out of proportion to the external cause, and without help, could lead to serious dysfunction.

In this chapter, we'll take a close look at depression—at what it is, and what it is not. I will discuss the symptoms that may be experienced by the depressed individual, and I'll explain the different categories of depression. Included is a self-quiz that will help you determine if you are depressed.

SYMPTOMS OF DEPRESSION

Unlike a passing blue mood, depression can totally absorb the mind and body, affecting the way one feels about oneself and the world. Moreover, depression is a sign of neither personal weakness nor self-indulgence. Depressed people cannot merely "pull themselves together." Without treatment, symptoms can last for weeks, months, or even years.

Symptoms of depression vary among and even within individuals. Sadness may not always be the dominant feeling. Depression can also be experienced as a numb or empty feeling, or perhaps as no feeling at all, positive or negative. Those who can't experience any sustained pleasure have a condition called *anhedonia*, literally meaning "absence of pleasure." Some depressed people experience extreme despair when they sense criticism, yet feel fine when they are accepted and included by others. A significant depressive disorder can range from brief and mild, to long-term and very severe—even life-threatening.

People suffering from depression may seek relief in a variety of ways, ranging from relatively harmless activities, such as shopping or changing jobs, to self-destructive behaviors, such as using alcohol or drugs. They may even injure themselves to take their minds off their inner pain. While some depressed persons seek out friends or family members for comfort, others prefer solitude.

The symptoms of depression include:

- Persistent sad, anxious, or "empty" mood
- Pessimism or feelings of hopelessness

- Loss of interest or pleasure in usual activities, including sex
- Insomnia, early-morning awakening, or excessive sleeping
- Agitation
- Decreased energy, fatigue, or a sense of being "slowed down"
- Low self-esteem, feelings of worthlessness, or excessive or inappropriate guilt
- Difficulty in concentrating, remembering, or making decisions
- Recurrent thoughts of death or suicide, a suicide attempt, or a specific suicide plan

Let's take a closer look at three significant symptoms: feelings of worthlessness or guilt, sleep disorders, and suicidal thoughts. (To check whether or not you are depressed, see "Testing Yourself for Depression—And Knowing When to Seek Help" on page 20.)

Sense of Worthlessness or Guilt

Often, depressed people suffer from feelings of inadequacy and self-loathing, despite their accomplishments. Corinne is a good example.

> *Corinne, a beautiful and gifted 32-year-old actress, was sure that she was a fraud. Her greatest fear was that "they'll find out how dumb and incompetent I really am." She was also terrified of getting old and losing her looks, certain that her other attributes were nonexistent. In fact, in addition to her acting career, Corinne had also written and directed a play, and was well respected in the theatrical community. She was still not convinced of her worth, however, and insisted, "It was a fluke."*

Testing Yourself for Depression—And Knowing When to Seek Help

For each question, circle the answer that comes closest to describing the way you feel. After you are finished, add up the numbers.

None or a little of the time	Some of the time	Good part of the time	Most or all of the time

1. I feel downhearted, blue, and sad.

1	2	3	4

2. I feel worse in the morning.

1	2	3	4

3. I have crying spells, or feel like it.

1	2	3	4

4. I have trouble sleeping through the night.

1	2	3	4

5. My appetite is poor.

1	2	3	4

6. I feel unattractive and not likable.

1	2	3	4

7. I am losing weight without trying.

1	2	3	4

8. I prefer to be alone.

1	2	3	4

9. I feel fearful.

1	2	3	4

10. I feel tired.

1	2	3	4

11. I have trouble concentrating.

1	2	3	4

12. It is an effort to do the things I used to do.

  1   **2**   **3**   **4**

13. I am restless and can't keep still.

  1   **2**   **3**   **4**

14. I feel hopeless about the future.

  1   **2**   **3**   **4**

15. I am irritable.

  1   **2**   **3**   **4**

16. I find it difficult to make decisions.

  1   **2**   **3**   **4**

17. I feel that I am not needed.

  1   **2**   **3**   **4**

18. My life feels empty and pointless.

  1   **2**   **3**   **4**

19. I feel that others would be better off if I were dead.

  1   **2**   **3**   **4**

20. I do not enjoy the things I used to enjoy.

  1   **2**   **3**   **4**

If your score is:

Below 30	You are within the normal range
Between 30 and 49	You are minimally to mildly depressed
Over 50	You are moderately to markedly depressed

If the quiz results indicate that you may be depressed, or if you are experiencing suicidal thoughts, speak to your internist or health practitioner first to rule out a physical cause for your problems. If necessary, your doctor should be able to refer you to a psychiatrist, preferably one with an orthomolecular orientation—that is, one who uses natural rather than manufactured substances whenever possible. Otherwise, in addition to a therapist, be sure to consult a naturopath or other natural medicine practitioner to look for an underlying chemical imbalance.

I understood Corinne's fear and loneliness. The frightened child inside, a victim of childhood abuse, still felt that she "must have deserved the mistreatment" that she had received at the hands of her disturbed mother. Our work consisted of helping Corinne find her own inner good mother, and to nurture her back to good mental health and a positive self-image.

People who, like Corinne, lack a sense of self-worth seem to have an Inner Critic looking over their shoulder, telling them how stupid, boring, ugly, and useless they are. They expect failure and rejection in whatever they do. When things do not turn out perfectly, they hear their Critic say, "See, I told you were incompetent (or useless, or worthless)." Depressed people often set impossible standards of performance for themselves. Then, when they can't meet these standards, the vicious cycle of negative self-worth is reinforced. The cycle can continue to build until it envelops the depressed individual in a prison of pessimistic thinking.

Treatment consists of the therapist actually addressing this Inner Critic, and offering it some understanding. This technique, called Voice Dialogue, was developed by Dr. Hal Stone and Dr. Sidra Stone, and has been an important tool in my practice (see *Embracing Your Inner Critic*, Appendix A).

Sleep Disorders

Depressed individuals frequently have sleep disorders. The most common one is waking up in the wee hours of the morning and not being able to get back to sleep. Then there are those depressed individuals who sleep too much, often spending most of the day in bed when they can. Such *hypersomnia* may be a sign that the depression is advanced and requires professional treatment. However, medical causes should be ruled out first.

There are a number of illnesses and metabolic imbalances that could lead to excessive sleep. Laura is a good example.

> *Laura was a troubled 16-year-old who, during my internship, was referred for evaluation to the psychiatric unit where I worked. Laura's symptoms included withdrawal, low self-esteem, and hypersomnia. She was overweight and didn't want to go to school, where she was doing poorly.*
>
> *In doing the initial physical examination, I noticed that one of Laura's eyes was slightly bulging. I asked if she had headaches, which she did. This would not be unusual in depression. However, I referred her to the neurology department for a brain scan. She turned out to have a brain tumor, which fortunately was benign and operable. Most of her symptoms were due to the tumor, and cleared up with her recovery from the surgery.*

While Laura had reasons to be depressed, her problem was in fact a physical one, and psychotherapy would not have been the appropriate treatment.

Recurrent Thoughts of Death or Suicide Attempts

Between 5 and 15 percent of severely depressed people take their lives each year. While most of them keep their thoughts to themselves until they commit the act, others actually do talk about it to friends and family members. Relatives and friends need to take threats of suicide seriously, and not see them as mere attention-getting devices. Anyone who has had suicidal thoughts should muster the courage to ask for help. Depression is a treatable disorder. Death is not.

Often, a suicidal person needs to be convinced that

the desire to die is a temporary state. He or she needs a trusted advisor to say, "Believe me, you can overcome your despair, and one day be glad that you didn't give in to your impulse to end it all." That advisor might be a therapist or psychiatrist; a minister, priest, or rabbi; a friend; or, in a moment of despair, a suicide hot line volunteer.

CLASSIFYING DEPRESSION

In conventional psychiatry, diagnosis falls into specific categories. The *Diagnostic and Statistical Manual of Mental Disorders* (*DSM-IV*, 1994) is a clinical guide that helps describe and categorize mental disorders. It was first developed in 1952 by a special committee of the American Psychiatric Association, which continues to update it.

Each revision of the *DSM* reflects the results of current research data, as well as the political and social climate. Some considerations come from society at large. For example, homosexuality was removed as a diagnosis, as was reference to individuals as "schizophrenic" or "alcoholic." These last terms were replaced by descriptive phrases, such as "an individual with schizophrenia" or " an individual with alcohol dependence." The idea is to label the disorders, not the people who suffer from them.

Other considerations come from within the mental health profession itself. The *DSM* is used by clinicians and researchers who follow many different schools of thought, including biological, psychodynamic, cognitive, behavioral, interpersonal, and family/systems. Each school has its own views regarding the origin of mental disorders. For example, depression can be attributed to everything from early emotional deprivation to an imbalance in brain chemistry, depending on the orientation of the examiner.

A significant statement in the introduction to the *DSM-IV* emphasizes that to make a distinction between "mental" and "physical" disorders is an outdated simplification that ignores the intimate connection between the mind and the body. It goes on to say, "There is an important physical dimension to mental disorders, and an important mental dimension in physical disorders. . . . The problem raised by the term 'mental' disorders has been much clearer than its solution and unfortunately, the term persists in the title of *DSM-IV* because we have not found an appropriate substitute."

This statement also reflects my own views. An imbalance in body and brain chemistry can cause many conditions, both mental and physical. As an orthomolecular psychiatrist, I do not think that classification by signs and symptoms accurately reflects how a patient will respond to treatment. Many "serious" depressions turn around fairly quickly when diagnosed according to the underlying deficiency or toxicity. The more we understand the mind-body connection, the easier it is to treat mental disorders.

Despite their limitations, the *DSM* classifications provide a good starting point when discussing the various types of depression. The *DSM-IV* classifies depression into several main groups:

- Major depressive disorder

- Dysthymia

- Adjustment disorder with depressed mood

- Bipolar disorder

- Seasonal affective disorder (SAD)

Let's take a closer look at these classifications, keeping in mind that they are merely guidelines, and not hard-and-fast labels. It is also important to remember that, as

I've said, mental disorders can result from a variety of physical disorders (see Chapter 3).

Major Depressive Disorder

Major depressive disorder is a serious depression that interferes with normal functioning. The standard psychiatric treatments for major depressive disorder include medication and psychotherapy. Electroconvulsive therapy (ECT), though seemingly radical, has been an effective treatment in difficult cases. However, simpler interventions are preferable and may be just as successful.

Arthur, a 70-year-old retired engineer brought to me by a worried daughter, is a typical example of someone with a major depressive disorder.

> *"Since Mom died, my father has totally disintegrated. It's been two years and, if anything, he seems to be getting worse. I know he misses her. They were so close. But shouldn't he be getting back to normal by now? Other members of the family have died, but it seems like their partners get on with their lives after a year or so."* She was correct: the usual mourning period is closer to one year. She described Arthur sitting at home alone, day after day, dozing in front of the television. Both the social isolation and excessive drowsiness are typical of this disorder. *"If I didn't bring him food, he would starve to death. He won't shop for food, even take-out, let alone cook. He's lost so much weight, and looks so pale, I'm really concerned for his health!"*
>
> Arthur was enveloped in a dark cloud of sadness. It was almost painful to be near him. He was disheveled and stared down at the ground, unable to make eye contact. When I asked how he was feeling, he tearfully responded, *"How should I feel? Why should I live? It's not worth living without my Betty. It should have been me that went, not her."*

Arthur and his wife had done every thing together. They raised a family of three children, then shared a home in a retirement community until her death from cancer. Arthur's physical health had been fairly good. He was on a low dose of medication for high blood pressure, but was not taking it regularly. In fact, when I checked his pressure, it was only slightly elevated. I was not concerned about a possible drug side effect in his case. Medication for high blood pressure can cause depression, but the dose was low and his use, erratic.

Arthur exhibited most of the signs and symptoms of a major depressive disorder. His was not a normal grief reaction, since it had gone on so long, and rather than improving, his condition was getting worse. It is important for depressed people and those who love them to understand that when a depression is this serious, professional help is necessary. Depression such as Arthur's can be life-threatening. If nothing else, he could simply have starved to death.

Arthur was a candidate for antidepressant medication, which I prescribed for him, along with a supply of nutritional supplements. I also gave him an injection of vitamin B_{12}, which is often deficient in the elderly, especially if they are malnourished. Too low a level of vitamin B_{12} can cause all the symptoms of depression (see Chapter 8). Replenishing the supply can do wonders, and in a short time, too.

I referred Arthur to a special therapy group for widows and widowers to help him deal with his grief, and to provide him with the emotional and social support he so badly needed. He made some friends in the group, began to socialize, and gradually emerged from the depths of his depression. After a few months, he would actually tell jokes when he came in to see me!

With the cooperation of his internist, Arthur gradually was able to discontinue use of his blood pressure medication, since the supplements were sufficient to control his pressure. I weaned him off antidepressant medication after six months, as I introduced St. John's wort, one 300-milligram capsule three times daily. The transition was no problem, and Arthur continued to feel and do well on a full nutrient support program.

Dysthymia

The term *dysthymia* comes from the Greek and literally means "bad mood." Though not as severe and disabling as a major depressive disorder, for those suffering from dysthymia, or mild to moderate depression, life is mostly "just going through the motions." They may be able to function at work or school, and possibly not even realize they are depressed. The disorder can start during childhood or can begin later in life. In most cases, it is chronic, or long-term, in nature, as we see in the case of Jodi.

> A 26-year-old bookkeeper, Jodi had been quiet, shy, and withdrawn most of her life. High school had been particularly rough, since she'd had no social life. She did not know how to "fit in." Nothing ever felt quite right. She couldn't understand what people meant by "just having a good time." When Jodi came to see me several years ago, referred by a concerned relative, she reported that it was "harder and harder to get up in the morning. I can't face the world. I just want to sleep—and eat." She was twenty pounds overweight, which definitely showed on her 5'2" frame. "I have never fit in, I don't know how other people seem to know what to do. You are my last hope."

Jodi began to work on her issue of self-esteem—she had none. In addition, I gave her some supplements.

Finally, after several diagnostic tests, I added a low dose of thyroid hormone, which was gradually increased to a proper level (see Chapter 8). This boosted her energy level and began to raise her low mood. She even started to exercise in the morning, something she had never done before.

After approximately six weeks, seeing there was still room for improvement, I added St. John's wort to Jodi's regimen, 300 milligrams twice daily. It was the icing on the cake. Two weeks later, we increased the dosage to three times daily. Within three weeks, she felt like a new person. "I actually feel normal," she exclaimed. In addition, her ability to focus and remember improved markedly, and she was better able to recall and use what she was learning in psychotherapy. Freed from the shyness that had previously pervaded her social life, she began to date. The last time I saw her, Jodi was working at a job she loved and had a steady boyfriend, Carl, with whom she was enjoying "just hanging out."

In almost all the cases I see, the patient's problems include a mixture of the psychological and the physical, and this mind-body connection is also inherent in the solutions. Jodi's typical dysthymia, consisting of depressed mood, low energy, weight gain, feelings of hopelessness, and low self-esteem, responded well to psychotherapy, thyroid medication, and St. John's wort.

Adjustment Disorder With Depressed Mood

Adjustment disorder, sometimes referred to as *reactive depression*, is a depression resulting from an identifiable stressor that has occurred within the preceding three months, such as the loss of a job, a divorce, or a disaster, such as an earthquake or fire. It impairs the individual's functioning in school or on the job, and also affects his or her relationships. The depression fades with time, generally within six months.

Reaction to the death of a loved one can also fall into this category. Such a loss may cause a full depressive syndrome, with associated symptoms such as poor appetite, weight loss, and insomnia. While the duration of "normal" bereavement varies considerably among different cultural groups, prolonged and marked depressive symptoms beyond two months, according to the *DSM-IV,* suggest the development of a major depressive disorder, as we saw in Arthur's case (see page 26).

Obviously, some people are more resilient than others. Early trauma often sets the stage for increased vulnerability to future traumatic events. Standard treatment can employ either psychotherapy or medication, and often a combination of the two is most effective.

It is important to discern whether a change in mood or personality is due primarily to an internal cause such as a chemical imbalance, as in Jodi's case, or to an external cause, as in the case of Ellen.

A 32-year-old single computer programmer, Ellen worked at a job she enjoyed, only to find out one day that she had acquired the Boss from Hell. Her old supervisor had been promoted, and a new person, a woman only slightly older than herself, was now in charge. They just did not get along. Ellen found herself increasingly frustrated, anxious, and depressed. At work, she was not her cheerful, productive self. She found herself on edge, ready to burst into tears at the least provocation. After work, she felt too tired to go out with friends and once she got home, she avoided phone calls. Ellen also had trouble sleeping, tossing and turning much of the night, awakening frequently with troubling dreams and anxious thoughts. This left

her exhausted the next morning, and even less moti-
vated to get up and go to work.

Ellen was showing typical signs of an adjustment disorder in response to an actual problem, as opposed to
a perceived problem. In her favor was the fact that she
had no prior history of depression.

With the help of supportive friends who did not give
up trying to get through to her, Ellen came out of her
depression. She decided to leave her job and to move
on in her career. While there was some stress involved
in the transition, she knew she had made the right
choice. Her old *joie de vivre* returned. Once again, she
was socializing, enjoying both her daily activities *and* her
new job.

Had Ellen felt the need to live with a bad situation,
perhaps because she was "destined to suffer" or "could
not control her life," this might have indicated a deeper-
seated psychological cause, such as unresolved issues
with power and authority. Had she had earlier experiences of being manipulated or abused by someone in
power, she might have been sensitized and less likely
to emerge from her depression as readily as she did.
Often people in Ellen's situation seek therapy and become stronger for it. In her case, she was rescued by
good friends who were insightful and caring enough to
support her until she saw the light.

Bipolar Disorder

Far less common than other forms of depressive disorders, *bipolar disorder* or *manic-depressive illness* involves cycles of depression and elation, or *mania*. Sometimes the
mood switches are dramatic and rapid, but most often,
they are gradual.

When in the depressed cycle, the bipolar person can

have any or all of the symptoms of a major depressive disorder (see page 26). During the manic cycle, he or she may experience any or all of the symptoms of mania. These include inappropriate elation or irritability; severe insomnia; grandiose notions and poor judgment; increased speech, energy, and sexual desire; disconnected and racing thoughts; and inappropriate social behavior. A milder form of elation, called *hypomania,* may replace the blatantly manic phase. The person may seem entertaining and fun, and even be creative and productive. The depressive part of the cycle, however, can be severe.

As we can see in Maggie's case, bipolar disorder often runs in families.

Just last week my patient Maggie called, saying she was afraid it was "one of those times again." Ordinarily enthusiastic and energetic, every six months or so this 52-year-old publicist begins to have difficulty getting up in the morning, doesn't want to exercise, and finds her work and life in general "just too much to handle." After several years of these cycles, she now recognizes the signs and comes in to see me. I step up her treatment regimen of medication, vitamins, and herbs. This will generally do the trick, and within a week or so, her mood and energy begin to return to normal. It is as if her depression were run by an internal time clock. Her mother and sister also have this same built-in program of mood swings.

Cyclothymic disorder is a milder form of bipolar disorder. Cyclothymic individuals have moderate mood swings that can go on for years. These emotional variations are not severe enough to be considered either major depression or full mania, but they can significantly interfere with a person's life.

A depressed bipolar individual may become manic when prescribed an antidepressant drug. This makes the use of St. John's wort a possible substitute, although there is insufficient clinical information to support its use. Some professionals believe that St. John's wort is *not* the treatment of choice, for fear that it may actually induce mania. However, despite the lack of clinical studies, it is used all the time in Germany with no problems. As in Maggie's case, I have used it in these situations, but with great care. More research needs to be done in this area before psychiatry can give a definite answer.

Seasonal Affective Disorder (SAD)

Another form of depression is *seasonal affective disorder* (SAD). This disorder is especially prevalent in countries at the extreme northern and southern latitudes, where there is only an hour or two of sunlight each day during the winter months. Sunlight deprivation triggers biochemical changes in the brain, resulting in a disturbance in the *circadian rhythm*, the natural cycles of the body that control sleeping, wakefulness, and hormone secretion. A disturbed circadian rhythm leads to such symptoms as marked decrease in energy, increased need for sleep, and carbohydrate craving. Yet, when affected individuals get their required dose of sunlight, they feel energetic and ready to get on with life. (For more information, see Chapter 4.)

As we've seen in this chapter, feeling depressed is not necessarily the same as suffering from clinical depression. A diagnosis of depression can only be made if a person displays a number of symptoms for a certain length of time, and only after physical causes have been ruled out. Anyone, however, who suffers from severe symptoms of depression, such as suicidal thoughts, should seek professional help without delay.

While the technical classifications of depression help a psychiatrist make a diagnosis, they do not explain the root causes of depression. As an orthomolecular psychiatrist, I believe these causes lie within the body's chemical makeup. I will explain this concept in the next chapter.

3

The Mind, the Body, and Mental Health

In view of the intimate connection between things physical and mental, we may look forward to the day when paths of knowledge will be opened up, leading from organic biology and chemistry to the field of neurotic phenomena.

Sigmund Freud

One out of every five people is affected by depression at some time in life, according to a recent study. Nearly 50 percent of the people between the ages of eighteen and fifty-four met the criteria for at least one of fourteen serious psychiatric illnesses. The elderly, who were not included in this particular study, have an even higher incidence of mental illness. And all evidence points to increasing rates of depression for people of all ages.

Why are so many people depressed? There are several reasons, since this disorder has several components. The best approach is one that takes into account all possible causes. In this chapter, we'll first look at the wholistic view of mental health, and how it differs from the conventional view. I'll then discuss the main components of depression.

A WHOLISTIC VIEW OF MENTAL HEALTH

Western medicine, and Western thought in general, presumes a division between the mind and body. This split grew out of eighteenth-century Enlightenment beliefs in science and reason as the sources of truth. These beliefs laid the foundation for the development of two distinct branches of medicine, one for physical illness and one for mental illness. If the physical cause of an illness is not readily apparent, it is usually considered to be mental, or psychosomatic, in origin.

Yet this antiquated view of the human body overlooks the clear interconnection of these two aspects. In fact, the "mind-body" is inseparable. Thanks to such modern-day teachers as Deepak Chopra, this truth has become more readily accepted: "Every time there is an event in the mind, there is a corresponding event in the body. . . . this interconnectedness is accomplished at a place sandwiched between mind and body, where thought turns into matter." The body works as an integrated whole, so trauma and stress, whether mental or physical, affect all systems. The more we know about the mechanisms of this connection, the better control we can have over our moods and our overall health.

On the most obvious level, we know that our bodies can suffer physical traumas that affect our mental health. Jerry is a good example. When Jerry, an electrician, fell off a ladder and broke his leg, the immediate pain was followed by weeks of discomfort and disability. His normally active life was seriously curtailed. He could not take his daily run, or even walk, and needed help simply getting up and down from his chair. Not surprisingly, Jerry became depressed. As his fracture healed and he become more mobile, his mood improved. By the time he resumed his usual activities, his depression had vanished. If we could have seen inside Jerry's brain, we would have noticed a definite shift in his brain chemistry reflecting these changes in mood.

This mind-body interaction works the other way, as well. When we feel depressed or stressed, there are often accompanying physical symptoms, such as headaches, unexplained back pain, or digestive problems. The expression "worrying yourself sick" can mean just that. Take Marlene, for example. She suffered constant illness and missed time from a receptionist job she disliked. Yet when she landed a desired job as a film production assistant, she became quite healthy, and her attendance, perfect. Her immune system had reflected her unhappiness, and became stronger as she became happier.

So how does depression develop? As we saw in Chapter 2, there are many schools of thought in psychiatry and psychology, each with its own ideas on the origin of depression, be it genetic, psychological, or biochemical. There is good evidence that all three of these factors interact with each other.

DEPRESSION: THE GENETIC FACTOR

Many diseases have a genetic component. So it is not surprising that research has shown a strong genetic component in depression. If you are depressed, there is a 25 percent chance that a first-degree relative—a parent, child, or sibling—is also depressed. If you are not depressed, the chance of this occurring is only 7 percent.

The best way to study this genetic influence is to study depression patterns in identical twins, especially those who have been reared apart through adoption. By definition, these twins share the exact same genetic material. Though raised in totally different environments, research has shown that if one twin becomes depressed, the other has a 40 to 70 percent chance of also becoming depressed, depending on which study you read. Meanwhile, their biologically unrelated siblings, raised in the same environment, do not share the same incidence, nor do fraternal (nonidentical) twins or other siblings—the correlation rates range from 0 to 13 percent. All of this proves the existence of a strong genetic component in depression.

The genetic component of depression interacts with the other components. For example, low brain levels of a chemical called serotonin, which is created from an amino acid called tryptophan, have been linked to depression (see page 46). In one interesting experiment, when research subjects were deprived of brain serotonin by feeding them a diet low in tryptophan, only those with a personal or family history of depression became depressed.

A genetic predisposition towards illness does not mean that the illness is inevitable. It's true that you cannot change your genetic inheritance. However, you can affect the way this inheritance is expressed. For example, you may very well have a genetic predisposition towards depression. That doesn't mean you *must* become depressed, as we saw from the twin studies—notice that the rate wasn't 100 percent.

DEPRESSION: THE PSYCHOLOGICAL FACTOR

What about the contributions of environment, early experiences, and trauma to depression? Research has clearly shown that not only will certain stressors cause depression as a direct response, but they may predispose an individual to future episodes of depression. Actual chemical changes occur in the brain in response to trauma, making the person more vulnerable to such future events, in addition to any genetic predisposition.

Researcher and author Candace Pert's work has

brought together many complex ideas regarding the mind-body connection. Pert has reported on some intriguing research done with baby monkeys. Similar to humans in their emotional responses, monkeys become depressed when separated from their mothers. If they are not being touched or held consistently, they become listless and withdrawn, show none of the usual primate social behavior, and demonstrate all the signs we associate with depression. In one research project, a number of depressed orphan monkeys were taken in by a "good mother" monkey who assumed the maternal nurturing role, in which she held and touched them constantly. Not only did these depressed little patients rally, but their brain chemistry showed corresponding changes. Here is a clear demonstration that the mind-body interaction is not a one-way street. (See *Molecules of Emotion* in Appendix A.)

A lack of love and support can also leave its marks on human children. Many children experience abuse on numerous levels every day of their lives. This may not be actual physical abuse, but psychological abuse, from overt bullying to subtle shaming, criticism, and lack of emotional support. According to Peter Levine in *Waking the Tiger Within*, such abuse produces changes in the brain that can lead to depression (see Appendix A).

Human experience provides still more evidence of the mind-body connection. Perhaps you are familiar with the problems of war veterans who suffer from Post Traumatic Stress Disorder (PTSD). They are generally depressed, anxious, and irritable. They have sleep disturbances, a variety of physical complaints, and difficulties in maintaining jobs and relationships. How does this happen? The trauma of sustaining injuries, of seeing their comrades die violent deaths while they survived, or of killing an enemy, soldier or civilian, makes an indelible mark on their brains. Their ability to maintain emotional balance is destroyed, and their lives become increasingly difficult.

Combat is far from the only experience that can lead to PTSD. Sarah is a good example.

Sarah was a 23-year-old graduate student who had been in a serious car accident one year prior to seeing me. She had suffered a broken pelvis and numerous other injuries when the car she was driving was hit broadside by a drunk driver. After that, her life was in shambles. Although her physical injuries had healed, she could not seem to get back on track. She could not complete her school assignments and was unable to keep her part-time job in the university library. Her attention span was short, she had trouble sleeping, and she was plagued by nightmares. She was also fatigued most of the time. Sarah was afraid to drive, and had to take public transportation, not an easy feat in Los Angeles. She confided that she felt her life was not worth living. Her strongest recollection of the accident was of being trapped—helpless and terrified. Her car had been so severely damaged that it had taken some time for rescue personnel to free her.

I was able to help Sarah by using Eye Movement Desensitization and Reprocessing (EMDR). Developed by psychologist Francine Shapiro, this technique helps an individual to recall a traumatic incident and reexperience the trauma, but in a safe setting. EMDR allows the mind to finally release suppressed emotions.

I asked Sarah to focus on the scene of being trapped, and on the feelings it brought up, both emotionally and physically. I then asked her to follow my fingers with her eyes in a rapid back-and-forth motion. She soon was in tears, recalling further details of the accident. We persisted with the eye movements, and another memory arose, one of an attempt by an adolescent boy, a neighbor, to sexually molest an eight-year-old Sarah. She had not thought of this scene in years, if ever. However, the theme was the same: "I'm trapped, helpless." She recalled feeling ashamed and guilty, somehow accepting blame for this incident. As we continued, I asked her to consider, as an adult, whose fault it was. From this new perspective, the answer was obvious. "Of course, I was just a kid. It was his fault. He was older." She visibly relaxed.

As our sessions continued, Sarah realized that she had lived under the shadow of the helplessness and guilt engendered by the attempted molestation without even realizing it. The car accident, though traumatic in itself, was more so because it fit into this old pattern. The end result was that Sarah regained her former capabilities and was able to continue with her life. Often it is not until a traumatic event occurs that one has the opportunity to recall and repair old wounds.

How could a fifteen-year-old incident affect someone so profoundly? The attempted molestation put Sarah's emotional memory bank, like an inner recorder or VCR, on pause. EMDR, which induces rapid eye movements, allowed her "VCR" to release, moving through the old film and into the present. A possible explanation for this is that the rapid eye movement of EMDR is similar to that which occurs during dream sleep. Emotional leftovers of the day are processed neatly by our brains through our dreams, and EMDR seems to be a way of producing the same healing function. Preliminary research indicates that corresponding changes in brain chemistry occur as a result of therapy. The attempted molestation could have affected Sarah's brain chemistry, leaving her more vulnerable to future trauma.

As in Sarah's case, symptoms may be evidence of buried information that can haunt an individual until it is uncovered and processed. The idea of treating symptoms alone, without looking underneath for the root cause, is shortsighted and, ultimately, not effective. During my years of practice, I have found that the best way to help patients deal with a difficult feeling is to encourage them to go right into it, embrace it, see what is behind it. Much of the pain we experience, including depression, can actually be a result of our attempts to resist it! We may reflexively try to shut out emotional pain. But that only forces it underground, haunting us in disguise as depression, anxiety, headaches, even serious illness. The solution? Instead of seeing painful feelings—or illnesses—as enemies, see them as messages from the unconscious mind and even the body.

Ignoring or turning off such signals can be a dangerous thing. It would be like unplugging a smoke alarm when it starts to ring. When the alarm goes off, we all know to look for the fire—or for the faulty wiring that's the source of the smoke. Depression and other apparently psychological symptoms can signify an unresolved psychological issue, but they can also be the result of a brain chemistry imbalance or a medical illness.

DEPRESSION: THE BIOCHEMICAL FACTOR

We can approach the biochemical agents of depression from two vantage points. One involves physical disorder and its effects on mental health, and the other involves the chemistry of the brain itself.

Physical Illness and Depression

Good health depends on both a healthy body and a healthy mind. Therefore, it is senseless to expect the brain to work correctly without the rest of the body being in proper balance. Every disorder or deficiency in the body affects the brain, which is extremely sensitive to imbalances caused by such physical problems as low blood sugar, water retention, or oxygen deprivation. Many people who don't respond well to psychotherapy show accelerated improvement once their conditions are properly diagnosed and treated.

The importance of the mind-body connection has not always been recognized, sometimes resulting in tragic consequences. For example, I recall learning in medical school about cretinism. Severely retarded from birth, people who suffered from cretinism were doomed to lives of miserable dependency, often in crowded institutions. Finally, it was discovered that they had been born with a deficiency of thyroid hormone due to a lack of iodine in the food their mothers ate during pregnancy. Since these patients did not receive the needed mineral in the womb, their thyroid glands could not develop normally, leading to retardation and other symptoms. The solution? Iodized salt, now a legislated dietary supplement! Was this illness inborn, genetic, and unchangeable? No. Cretinism was simply not recognized as a mineral deficiency, and could not be correctly treated until the dietary link was discovered.

Another example of a physical illness masquerading as a mental illness is pellagra. During the nineteenth and early twentieth centuries, mental institutions were filled with pellagra patients, who were quite demented. Eventually, it was discovered that this severe mental illness could be reversed—or better yet, prevented—through administration of niacin (vitamin B_3). Although pellagra is a physical disease, one of the first and most prominent symptoms is mental in nature. Once doctors recognized the disease's true origin, pellagra patients all but disappeared from mental hospitals.

Medicine continues to commit this type of error. In the 1950s, Dr. Abram Hoffer and Dr. Humphrey

Osmond, pioneers in the field of orthomolecular psychiatry, noticed that many people with schizophrenia responded well to high doses of niacin. The psychiatric establishment would not accept these remarkable findings, and soon the advent of the major tranquilizers left this discovery behind. While the pharmaceutical industry profited from these drugs, the root cause of and simple solution to many cases of schizophrenia were ignored. There are many conditions like this.

I believe that medical illness causes depression more often than many doctors suspect, and hope the day comes when psychiatrists routinely look for underlying physical disorders. In my own practice, I prefer to begin psychotherapy only after excluding a physical cause, such as those listed in Table 3.1.

Since the mind and body together form a complex interactive system, several of these biological factors may occur at once. Imbalance in one area often leads to imbalance in another, requiring a careful sifting through the various signs and symptoms to arrive at a correct diagnosis and treatment. Nutritional imbalances will be covered in greater detail in Chapter 8.

Brain Chemistry and Depression

Regardless of the triggering factors, the underlying mechanism of depression is a shift in brain chemistry.

The brain is made up of nerve cells, or *neurons*. Between the neurons are small gaps called *synapses*. In order for a message to pass from one neuron to its neighbor across the synapse, a chemical messenger called a *neurotransmitter* is released. The *presynaptic neuron*—the one that is sending the message—produces the neurotransmitter, which moves toward the *postsynaptic neuron* on the receiving end. The neurotransmitter molecule is shaped like a key that will fit only a certain

Table 3.1. Possible Medical Causes of Depression

Category	Specific Conditions
Recognized medical conditions	Diabetes; liver disease; autoimmune disease, including rheumatoid arthritis, lupus, and multiple sclerosis; heart disease; high blood pressure; cancer
Medications	Blood pressure-lowering medications, especially beta-blockers; anti-inflammatories, such as cortisone; birth control pills; tranquilizers, such as Valium and Thorazine; interferon, used to treat hepatitis and certain cancers
Metabolic imbalances	Anemia; hypoglycemia (low blood sugar); premenstrual syndrome (PMS); food and chemical sensitivities
Nutritional deficiencies	The lack of vitamins, minerals, or amino acids, caused by poor diet, malabsorption, or anorexia
Hormonal imbalances	In pituitary, pineal, thyroid, adrenal, or sex hormones, or a combined imbalance
Toxins	Substances of abuse, especially withdrawal from stimulants such as caffeine, nicotine, and cocaine; heavy metals, including lead and mercury; chemicals, including petroleum products such as PCBs (used in making plastics, solvents, and pesticides)
Infections	Any systemic infection: fungal infections such as candida, viral infections such as Epstein-Barr virus and cytomegalovirus, Lyme disease

lock, called the *receptor site*, on the postsynaptic neuron. When the key slides into the lock, the message has been received, and the receptor is either activated or inhibited, depending on its function.

Once its job is complete, the neurotransmitter molecule is released back into the synapse. It might return to the precursor neuron, where it can be used again. Or it might remain in the synapse, where it floats around with other kinds of chemical messengers. The molecule may then continue the cycle by reconnecting with a receptor, or it may be inactivated by an enzyme such as monoamine oxidase (MAO).

Mood is affected by changes in the relative levels of various neurotransmitters. The question is, what causes these variations in neurotransmitter levels, and, conversely, can a change in mood alter the balance of our neurotransmitters?

Serotonin and Other Mood-Affecting Substances

One of the most important neurotransmitters is *serotonin*. Serotonin influences many physiological functions, including blood pressure, digestion, body temperature, and pain sensation. It also affects circadian rhythm, or the body's response to the cycles of day and night, as well as mood. Low levels of serotonin are associated with:

• Depression

• Obsessive thinking

• Anxiety

• Increased sensitivity to pain

• Emotional volatility, including violent behavior against self and others

• Alcohol and drug abuse

• Premenstrual syndrome (PMS)

- Increased sexual desire
- Carbohydrate cravings
- Sleep disturbances

On the other hand, healthy levels of serotonin are associated with emotional and social stability. In fact, Prozac is used to treat depression because it can raise serotonin levels.

Research supports the connection between high serotonin levels and positive mood. Michael Raleigh and Michael McGuire of UCLA studied vervet monkeys to explore the relationship between mood and status. They found that the highest ranking, or alpha, male in each group had the highest level of serotonin. When these males lost their alpha status, their serotonin levels plummeted, and they withdrew, much like the depressed baby monkeys we met on page 39. Meanwhile, by administering Prozac to a non-alpha male, Raleigh and McGuire were able to turn that individual into the new alpha monkey.

There are several factors that affect neurotransmitter levels and mood. One factor is diet. Neurotransmitters are made of amino acids, the building blocks of protein. Inadequate protein in the diet can reduce the availability of neurotransmitters, thus affecting mood. Neurotransmitter levels can also be affected by the presence of MAO, a neurotransmitter inactivator. Another influence involves the sensitivity level of the receptor site to the neurotransmitter.

Serotonin and other neurotransmitters are important mood-affecting chemicals, but they are certainly not the only ones. The sex hormones, such as estrogen and testosterone, affect brain cells directly. And there are the endorphins, naturally occurring substances similar in structure to morphine and heroin. Endorphins function like natural opiates in our brains, producing pleasurable

feelings such as "runner's high." Certain depressed people have low levels of endorphins. This is especially true
of those patients who cut or otherwise mutilate themselves.

The Stress Response and Depression

A further influence on mood involves the body's endocrine system, which produces hormones, substances
that regulate processes throughout the body. The *hypothalamus*, a part of the brain that serves as the command
center of the endocrine system, reacts to stress by sending a signal to the *pituitary gland*, the body's master
gland, which lies right beneath the hypothalamus. The
pituitary, in turn, signals the *adrenal glands*, which lie on
top of the kidneys, to release two hormones, adrenaline
and cortisol. *Adrenaline* is responsible for obvious physical effects such as increases in respiration, heart rate,
and blood pressure. *Cortisol* causes the liver to release
glucose into the bloodstream for quick energy. It also
depresses the immune system, enabling the body to use
all of its energy reserves in dealing with the emergency
at hand. This "fight-or-flight" response allows the body
to react to danger.

The hypothalamus-pituitary-adrenal chain of command
has served humans well for thousands of years as a
means of survival. In depressed people, however, this
process malfunctions. It appears that continual stress
early in life disrupts the cycle; instead of shutting off
once the crisis is over, this process continues, with the
hypothalamus continuing to signal the adrenals to produce cortisol. This increased cortisol production exhausts
the stress mechanism, leading to fatigue and depression.
Cortisol also interferes with serotonin activity, furthering
the depressive effect.

Moreover, continually high cortisol levels lead to sup-
pression of the immune system through increased pro-

duction of interleukin-6, an immune-system messenger. This coincides with research findings that stress and depression have a negative effect on the immune system. Reduced immunity makes the body more susceptible to everything from colds and flus to cancer. For example, the incidence of serious illness, including cancer, is significantly higher among people who have suffered the death of a spouse in the previous year.

Fortunately, this immune-suppression process can be corrected—with psychotherapy, medication, or any number of other positive influences that restore hope and a feeling of self-esteem. For example, this stress-depression cycle was reversed in the baby monkeys who received "hug therapy." And recent research shows that St. John's wort blocks the cortisol response by inhibiting interleukin-6, at least in the laboratory. The body's ability to recover from adversity is remarkable.

The difference between conventional and orthomolecular psychiatry lies, I believe, in the overall reluctance of the medical profession to look at deeper metabolic causes of illness in general and mental illness in particular. I have seen case after case of all kinds of illness underdiagnosed (read: misdiagnosed) because the imbalance that would be obvious to an orthomolecular physician was simply not found. If the doctor is unaware of the deeper connection between body chemistry and illness, he or she will never test for these elements, and the opportunity for healing is lost. Orthomolecular physicians, however, look further, aware that depression can be a signal that there's a malfunction in the mind-body continuum. In the next chapter, I'll explain how St. John's wort can help both the body and the mind.

4

St. John's Wort—
The Versatile Herb

It was never like this on Prozac . . . there's more laughter.

Kate, 48-year-old author

The herbalists of ancient times knew about the powers of St. John's wort, and they used it for a wide variety of ailments. However, Western medicine discarded the ancient knowledge, dropping the study of herbs from medical school curricula. In its assumption that the old teachings were unscientific old wives' tales, the medical profession lost touch with these gifts of the natural world.

In this chapter, we'll first look at the history of this fascinating plant. I'll then discuss St. John's wort's antidepressive effects and its numerous other benefits.

AN ANCIENT MEDICINE REDISCOVERED

St. John's wort presents a wonderful paradox. Known to healers for thousands of years, it has become an overnight sensation in the modern media. No doubt utilized by some of the earliest civilizations, the oldest records of its use come from Greek and Roman times, according to herbalist Christopher Hobbs. Dioscorides, the foremost Greek herbalist, recommended it for sciatica and malaria relief, and as a diuretic and female tonic. Pliny the Elder, the Roman naturalist, found it effective against snakebite when mixed with wine. (We're not sure whether the wine was to be mixed with the herb, or just drunk to take one's mind off the pain!)

The botanical name *Hypericum* comes from the Greek words *yper*, meaning upper, and *eikon*, or image. The Greeks and Romans believed that St. John's wort protected them from evil spirits and witches' spells, and often placed the herb in their homes and above statues of their gods. Perhaps the spirits and spells referred to depression and anxiety, mental disorders with no obvious physical cause.

The early Christians incorporated many ancient beliefs into their new religion. Preexisting spring rituals, for instance, were renamed as saints' feast days. In this tradition, Christian mystics named *Hypericum* after St. John the Baptist. It was traditionally collected on St. John's Day, June 24, and soaked in olive oil for days to produce a blood-red anointing oil, said to symbolize the blood of the saint.

By the thirteenth century, belief in the herb's mystical power was well established. People brought the flowers of the plant into their houses on Midsummer Eve, or St. John's Eve (June 23), to protect them from the powers of evil. In another common practice, they put the plants under their pillows on St. John's Eve. According to legend, the saint would appear in a dream, give his blessing, and protect the sleeper from dying during the following year. St. John's wort was also burned in bonfires on St. John's Eve to drive away evil spirits, purify the air, and protect crops.

According to the traditional doctrine of signatures, an

herb's physical appearance gives an indication of its specific healing power. Red plants, reminiscent of blood, were felt to be good for wound healing. The red oil in St. John's wort was no exception. Crusaders not only carried the plant to protect themselves from sorcery, but also used the soaked flowers and leaves as an ointment to help heal the wounds of battle. Physicians in the sixteenth century found the herb to be very effective for treating deep wounds. The first *London Pharmacopoeia*, published in 1618, recommended that the flowers be placed in oil and allowed to stand for three weeks. The resulting tincture was used for wounds and bruises. Other traditional folk uses for St. John's Wort include the treatment of gout, rheumatism, and jaundice.

When the first European colonists arrived in North America, they found that the Native Americans were already familiar with the herb. The latter used it for diarrhea, fevers, snakebite, and wounds and other skin problems. It later served as a valuable medicine for treating soldiers' wounds during the Civil War. St. John's wort was also prescribed by the homeopaths of the period for a variety of ailments, as it is to this day. (For a list of the active ingredients in St. John's wort and their effects, see "The Many Active Ingredients in St. John's Wort" on page 54.)

Unfortunately, toward the end of the nineteenth century, the medical establishment in the United States turned its back on traditional folk remedies. Teachings that had been passed down through the ages were dismissed as primitive superstition. Medical researchers considered most of the complex chemical constitution of a plant to be extraneous, and their objective was to isolate the plant's so-called "active ingredient." Now, of course, we realize these "extras" are often the ingredients that hold the secret to a plant's strength and healing power.

The Many Active Ingredients in St. John's Wort

While hypericin has received most of the attention in scientific research, there are other chemicals in St. John's wort that may contribute to its antidepressant effects. These ingredients have a number of additional properties, as well. Here are some of the herb's primary chemical constituents and their actions:

Amentoflavone (13′, 118-biapigenin)	Anti-inflammatory, antiulcerogenic
GABA	Sedative
Hyperforin	Antibacterial against gram-positive bacteria, wound healing; neurotransmitter inhibitor; potential anticarcinogenic
Hypericin	Antiviral
13, 118-biapigenin	Probably sedative
2-methyl-butenol	Sedative
Proanthocyanidins	Antioxidant, antimicrobial, antiviral, vasorelaxant
Pseudohypericin	Antiviral
Quercitrin	*In vitro* MAO inhibiting activity
Xanthones	Antidepressant, antimicrobial, antiviral, diuretic, cardiotonic, MAO inhibitor

---

This table is one of many found in an excellent resource, *St. John's Wort Monograph*, that summarizes the latest research on the herb. It is edited by Roy Upton of the American Herbal Pharmacopoeia (Box 5159, Santa Cruz CA 95063, website: herbal-ahp.org) and published by the American Botanical Council (see Appendix B) in *Herbalgram* no. 40, Summer 1997.

Medical authorities established what we now know as conventional medicine, focusing their attention on medical and surgical techniques, and manufactured drugs. They lobbied Congress and the state legislatures for the prohibition of herbal medicine, which had a chilling impact on the legitimate use of herbs to promote health. Current laws still restrict the use of specific healing claims on herbal medicine labels. Only recently has conventional medicine begun to explore once again the potential contributions that herbs can make to health. (See Chapter 5 for more information.)

ST. JOHN'S WORT AND DEPRESSION

Conventional medicine may be scratching its collective head about the value of St. John's wort, but that has not stopped ordinary people such as Kate from reaping its benefits, including its remarkable ability to fight depression.

Kate, a 48-year-old married author and public speaker, had a super-busy lifestyle, with frequent deadlines and an intense travel schedule, and it had caught up with her. "While on an impossible deadline, I had a total collapse. I was exhausted, stressed, and depressed. My doctor put me on Prozac, but it made me even more depressed, and then, I couldn't sleep. He gave me sleeping pills that zonked me, and that was it. I stopped the Prozac. Then I read about St. John's wort, and thought I'd try it, 250 milligrams twice daily. I figured it couldn't hurt! Three weeks later, my husband Mike suddenly noticed: 'You're different! You seem more relaxed, less tense. What's going on?'"

Kate hadn't told him she was taking St. John's wort, but her change in attitude was obvious. "One of the most dramatic things I began to notice is I felt happy and ebullient in the mornings, which I never was before. It was never like this on Prozac. I'm more energetic and focused, and there's more laughter!"

Her good news continued. "Our sex life has always been very sporadic and difficult. Four weeks after starting St. John's wort, we had a sexual experience that was distinctively different from any we have had in our twenty years together. I felt an openness, a sexuality, that was a pervasive feeling, coming from my very core. It was extraordinary for me, and Mike was just swept away. I don't think I'd ever felt that way, even when I was younger. And this openness has continued."

In a separate conversation with me, Mike was even more effusive than Kate. "I can't believe how she's changed. She's always been so tense, barely available, especially when she's stressed. Now, she's a delight. We are having the time of our lives!"

This all sounds too good to be true, you might say. Maybe it's an isolated incident, or simply the power of suggestion as a result of all the positive publicity surrounding St. John's wort. How representative is Kate? According to the research I have read, reports from other physicians and practitioners, and my own clinical experience—hers is not an isolated case.

In fact, one of my colleagues, a wholistic physician, had been asked by a woman in his yoga class what he knew about St. John's wort. He gave her what information he had. Two months later, she came running up to him in class, exclaiming, "I must thank you. The St. John's wort changed my whole life, my outlook, everything. It's like a veil lifted from around my head. I've never felt so good. And I'm dreaming again, and remembering my dreams. I can hardly believe it!"

Contemporary Research Proves the Value of St. John's Wort

In Germany, where herbal medicine is a standard part of the medical-school curriculum, 80 percent of German doctors prescribe herbs such as St. John's wort on a regular basis. Not suprisingly, a great deal of the research on this most valuble herb has been conducted in Germany.

Mild to moderate depressions respond well to treatment with St. John's wort. More than twenty studies involving thousands of patients confirm the herb's ability to reduce and often eliminate the symptoms associated with these conditions. Compared with both placebos—inert comparison substances—and various antidepressant drugs, St. John's wort has come out on top every time.

The herb's success rate as an effective antidepressant is between 60 to 80 percent, a rate equal to that of prescription drugs such as Prozac, with far fewer side effects. A drug monitoring study published in 1994 looked at the experiences of 3,250 patients who were treated with St. John's wort. It found that only 2.4 percent of these patients reported any side effects at all, a rather remarkable finding when you consider that Prozac produces side effects at least ten times more frequently, and that even the placebos produced side effects. (We will look at this and other studies in detail in Chapter 6.)

Scientists are not yet sure of exactly how St. John's wort works (see page 61). For example, a preliminary National Institute of Mental Health (NIMH) *in vitro,* or test tube, study indicates that St. John's wort has a high affinity for GABA receptor sites in the brain (see Chapter 3). The amino acid GABA (gamma-amino-butyric acid), plays a role in mood regulation: GABA levels are low in people with depression, and GABA-

enhancing agents show both antidepressant and an-
tianxiety effects. Despite the herb's Valium-like effect on
anxiety, there is a lack of sedation, which is an obvious
advantage in treatment.

Let's see how St. John's wort can help several specific problems.

Sleep Disorders and Insomnia

One of St. John's wort's major advantages over prescription antidepressant medications is its ability to
promote a better quality of sleep. Unlike St. John's
wort, most antidepressants lengthen the time it takes
to enter the REM (rapid eye movement) sleep phase,
reducing or even eliminating REM sleep. Far from in-
active during sleep, the subconscious mind is busy an-
alyzing the day's events and processing feelings during
the dreaming or REM phase. This is essential for mental health.

Pete is an example of someone whose sleep disorder
was relieved by a combination of St. John's wort and
sedating herbs.

> Pete, a 40-year-old businessman, blamed his inability to
> sleep on his stressful job. He would toss and turn, wor-
> rying about his work problems and about being too
> tired to handle them the next day. He was always ex-
> hausted from lack of sleep.
>
> Dreading the thought of another tormented night,
> Pete asked his family doctor for a sleeping pill pre-
> scription. Fortunately for him, his doctor was aware of
> natural alternatives, and suggested an herbal ap-
> proach to the problem. For the insomnia, he recom-
> mended an herbal combination of valerian and kava,
> both excellent sedating herbs, and for the underlying
> depression, St. John's wort. Pete was then able both to

get to sleep and to remain asleep through the night. Just having sufficient rest was enough to help his mood. Then, after a few weeks, the St. John's wort began to work more noticeably, and he could feel his mood lift further, and he had less need for the other herbs.

Had Pete gone the standard medical route, the requested sleeping pill prescription would have handled the symptom—temporarily. The downside would have been *habituation*, in which he would have needed increasing doses for the same result, in addition to the lack of REM sleep.

St. John's wort is also helpful for insomnia in general, not just that associated with depression. Prescription sedatives often produce grogginess or a hangover effect the next morning, and can also be addictive. St. John's wort, on the other hand, works with the body's own sleep-promoting mechanism to bring on restful sleep. It harmoniously enhances the natural actions of the brain, instead of drugging it into submission. Consequently, one awakens feeling more relaxed and refreshed. Since it can take a week or so for this effect to begin, St. John's wort is recommended mainly for recurring insomnia, and not just an occasional night of tossing and turning.

Seasonal Affective Disorder (SAD)

St. John's wort can also be used to treat SAD. As we saw in Chapter 2, persons with SAD, a form of major depression, are profoundly affected by the lack of sunlight that occurs in autumn and winter. This triggers biochemical changes in the brain, directed by the brain chemicals melatonin and serotonin, and leads to such symptoms as depression, impaired concentration, anxi-

ety, marked decrease in energy and libido, and carbohydrate cravings. Also, like bears preparing to hiber-
nate, these people eat more, gain weight, and need
more sleep.

Scientists have found *light therapy* to be effective in
treating SAD. Light therapy consists of exposing the individual to a set of full-spectrum fluorescent lights during the early morning and evening hours. Alternatively,
lighted visors can be worn that shine light through the
eyes and into the pineal gland. This stimulates the production of melatonin, a hormone associated with cyclic
bodily processes. St. John's wort can be combined with
light therapy for greater effect (see Chapter 6). In the
view of herbalist Terry Willard, the herb "brings light
into dark places." He finds it extremely effective in
treating the rampant SAD that occurs during the long,
dark winters of northern Canada, where he lives and
works.

Premenstrual Syndrome (PMS)

PMS is a common complaint that produces both physical and mental symptoms. Since some of its mental
symptoms are similar to those experienced during depression, including irritability, tension, and restlessness,
it should come as no surprise that St. John's wort can
help. For centuries, herbalists have recognized the herb's
value in treating discomforts associated with the menstrual cycle, and it remains a most widely utilized natural treatment for PMS, as well as menstrual cramps.
The latter is likely due to the herb's ability to reduce
uterine levels of *prostaglandins,* substances that can promote inflammation. You will often find women's tonics
that contain St. John's wort in combination with other
ingredients that function in a similar manner (see
Chapter 5).

What to Expect and When to Expect It

As with most antidepressants, it may take three or four weeks before you notice a significant effect. Larger dosages are unlikely to reduce this time lag. On the other hand, positive results often occur sooner. For example, within a week to ten days, many people notice improved sleep: better quality, fewer interruptions, and even more dreaming. After one to two weeks, there may be improvements in appetite, energy levels, and physical well-being. By the second or third week, there is a reduction in emotional symptoms, with less anxiety, a more positive mood, and a greater sense of peace.

Many of my patients report positive effects almost immediately, with a sensation in their brains of "a weight being lifted," decreased anxiety, and an enhanced ability to concentrate. We don't know if this is a "real" response, or simply a placebo effect brought on by positive expectations (see Chapter 6). It is also important to remember that as with any remedy, natural or synthetic, St. John's wort affects different people in different ways. Some people experience changes sooner or later than average, and some don't experience changes at all.

How does St. John's wort work? At this point, it is hard to give a definitive answer. While initially thought to be an MAO inhibator, St. John's wort is more likely similar in its action to the SSRIs such as Prozac (see Chapter 7). These reduce the rate at which the brain cells reabsorb serotonin, leaving more of the neurotransmitter molecules in the synapses, thereby enhancing receptor-site activity (see Chapter 3). And, as I've said before, in people who are depressed, the brain's receptor sites are often less sensitive than normal, and it is possible that the herb enhances the sensitivity of these sites. It has also been suggested that St. John's wort inhibits interlukin-6, a chemical messenger that mediates the stress response (see page 49). This gives St. John's wort an antistress effect.

In any case, do not expect instant results, like Rob did.

> Rob, an artist acquaintance of mine, was a moody, impulsive guy who, for example, would go from being excited about a project to forgetting about it entirely. He heard about St. John's wort, and thought it might smooth out his moods. He asked my opinion, and I agreed that it was worth a try. He began that very day. When he didn't feel any different an hour after his first capsule, he took another. And another. By the end of the day, he had taken four. Then he called me, asking why it wasn't working! I explained that St. John's wort was not a stimulant, nor was it rapid in its action. Rather, the antidepressant effects accumulate over time, and that he had to take it regularly for a few weeks before he would begin to notice a difference. Rob was disappointed.

Rob seemed to be caught up in the "take a pill for fast, fast relief" mentality.

Some depressions may not respond at all to St. John's wort, depending on the source of the depression. Take Gretchen, for example.

> Gretchen, a bright, creative hairstylist and artist, had been depressed for a couple of weeks. "I was going home at night and crashing, not wanting to see anyone. I just wanted to sleep when I wasn't working. I had read about St. John's wort, and decided to try it for two weeks. Nothing changed. Then I remembered that I have a tendency to be anemic." When her iron was low, Gretchen would feel tired and depressed. "I

*went off to the health food store, bought some iron,
took it daily, and within a week, was feeling normal."*

Was this a St. John's wort failure? I don't think so.
Rather, Gretchen is a great example of someone who un-
derstands her own body, looks for a recognizable pattern, and feels confident enough to take charge of her
own health when necessary. Before assuming that the
source of a depression is a neurotransmitter imbalance
(see Chapter 3), you should look for a nutritional deficiency or other physical disorder. We will look at this
in more detail in Chapter 8.

When there is a neurotransmitter imbalance, my preference is to start with St. John's wort, unless the case
is one of the exceptions mentioned in Chapter 3 (that
is, major depression or bipolar disorder). This herb still
has many advantages over the synthetic antidepressants.

ST. JOHN'S WORT'S EFFECTS
ON OTHER DISORDERS

Though current attention focuses on St. John's wort's
role in the treatment of depression, the herb has been
shown to have many other valuable medical uses as
well. Studies have shown that St. John's wort has broad
antiviral and antibacterial properties, and relieves inflammation. This confirms its traditional usage as an excellent treatment for wounds and burns. Also, St. John's
wort may be useful in cancer treatment.

How can one herb produce so many different benefits? St. John's wort is a complex mixture of at least ten
groups of active ingredients (see page 54), each with its
own effects. It works with our bodies to achieve healing in multiple ways. A manufactured drug, in contrast,
is aimed at one specific target, and often produces neg-

ative side effects when its action expands beyond that target. The opposite is true of herbs such as St. John's wort, which contain compounds that work together to accomplish more than any one component could do on its own. Rather than unwanted side effects, you receive bonus healing effects.

It is also important to remember, as we saw in Chapter 3, that the wholistic view of medicine does not separate illness into two neat stacks, physical ailments and mental ailments. To begin with, many physical disorders can lead to depression, and depression in turn can lead to physical illness. In addition, the mind-body continuum has common influences, and imbalances can be bodywide in nature. Therefore, the use of St. John's wort, by relieving your physical problems, may very well help lift your mood.

Antiviral Actions

St. John's wort has been shown to have dramatic antiviral activity, although in dosages much higher than those required to treat depression. Experiments, both in test tubes and in animals, have indicated that two of the active chemicals in the plant, hypericin and pseudo-hypericin, are clearly effective against a number of *retro-viruses*, including the herpes and hepatitis C viruses. The herbs show significant activity against influenza types A and B; the vesicular stomatitis virus, which causes inflammation of the mouth; and even the Epstein-Barr virus, which is associated with infectious mononucleosis and chronic fatigue syndrome.

Hypericin and pseudohypericin show great promise for several reasons. They inactivate or interfere with the ability of viruses to reproduce. They are also able to cross the *blood-brain barrier*, an organic safety mechanism that prevents many substances from reaching the brain.

Intended to filter out toxic substances, this barrier also denies entry to many beneficial ones. The ability to cross this barrier is particularly meaningful in dealing with viruses that target the brain.

In several cases, the two chemicals have proven effective in preventing disease after a single oral or intravenous dose. This is highly unusual, since viruses are normally much more resistant than that to treatment. Compared with other antiviral medications, St. John's wort has very few side effects, although there can be some phototoxicity, or extreme sensitivity to light, when it is administered in very high doses. Researchers are now studying the potential of hypericin against other viruses.

At New York University, Dr. Daniel Meruelo and Dr. Gad Lavie are researching the use of hypericin in fighting the human immunodeficiency virus (HIV), the virus associated with acquired immunodeficiency syndrome (AIDS). In mice, hypericin has been shown not only to inactivate the virus, but also to shield the membranes of healthy cells from attack. No other current antiviral drug is able to do this. It is also possible that hypericin, if added to donated blood, may protect transfusion recipients from becoming infected with HIV.

In Cooper and James's study of thirty-one AIDS patients, the researchers found a 13 percent increase in counts of T helper cells (T cells), an important component of the immune system, after one month of supplementation with St. John's wort. This higher level was maintained after four months. In a study by Stenbeck and Wernet, sixteen patients saw their counts of CD4, another immune-system component, either improve or remain stable when they took St. John's wort over a forty-month period. Only two of the sixteen developed the kinds of opportunistic infections that often affect people with faulty immune systems. These studies indicate that St. John's wort may very well play an important role in the fight against AIDS, and research is continuing in this area.

It is worth noting that, so far, the antiviral research has been done using refined synthetic hypericin, identical to natural hypericin but lacking the other medicinal compounds found in the whole herb. Unrefined St. John's wort extract has been shown clinically to have antiviral properties, but no study has yet been done comparing the two forms.

Wound-Healing and Antibacterial Actions

Several studies have confirmed the traditional use of St. John's wort in wound healing. Hyperforin and novoimanine, antibiotic chemicals found in the plant's flowers and leaves, are at least partly responsible for these antibacterial and healing properties. One German study showed that an ointment containing the herb reduced healing time dramatically and resulted in less scarring. First-degree burns healed within forty-eight hours, and third-degree burns healed three times faster without the usual formation of scar tissue.

A friend of mine verified St. John's wort's healing powers through personal experience. When her four-year-old son accidentally scalded his hand with boiling water, she immediately applied St. John's wort oil to the site. The pain ceased, and he stopped crying. The redness cleared in a few days, with none of the blistering or scarring that generally follows such a burn.

St. John's wort acts against a wide variety of bacteria. In one study, it was found to be more effective than the antibiotic sulfanilamide against the *Staphylococcus* (staph) bacteria responsible for many hospital epidemics. The bacteria that causes tuberculosis, the fungus *Candida*, and the gastrointestinal parasite *Shigella* have all responded to St. John's wort. These findings are particularly important because of the increasing incidence of antibiotic-resistant strains of bacteria.

Anti-Inflammatory and Immune-Enhancing Actions

St. John's wort has been used for centuries to reduce inflammation and to stimulate the immune system. Ointments containing the herb have been valuable tools for medics on the fields of battle until this century, when they were was replaced by synthetic drugs. It appears that the flavonoid component in the herb is the main anti-inflammatory agent, although others contribute to its immune-enhancing activity. Russian researchers recently discovered that this complex herb contains substances that both stimulate and suppress immunity. This allows St. John's wort to boost the ability of the immune system to fight infection, while at the same time decreasing the immune processes that promote inflammation in wounds and other injuries. Substances that can perform such balancing acts are called *tonics*, or adaptogens. A synthetic drug only has one active ingredient, so it simply can't manage such a harmonious balancing of the body's immune response. This is one of the main advantages of herbal remedies.

Someone who has learned about St. John's wort's immune-boosting powers is Renata.

Renata, a 38-year-old woman with severe chronic fatigue syndrome, was depressed and constantly exhausted. She consulted a doctor at a major university medical center, who simply recommended that she rest. Then, a clerk in a health food store suggested St. John's wort in 300-milligram capsules. Renata took a capsule twice a day before increasing her intake to three times a day. Within a few weeks, her depression lifted and her energy began to return. By six weeks, not only was she free of symptoms, but she noticed that she did not get her regular attack of herpes in conjunction with her period, a common occurrence in susceptible women. Moreover, a year later, Renata is still taking St. John's wort and remains completely symptom-free.

This case is a great illustration of St. John's wort's multiple functions. Renata's experience is particularly remarkable considering the usual difficulty in treating herpes. (For more information on chronic fatigue syndrome, see Chapter 8.)

St. John's Wort and Cancer

There is promising research showing that St. John's wort has anticancer effects. It also has been shown to be effective in preventing cell damage from radiation, including damage to delicate intestinal lining and bone marrow cells in test animals. I believe that if these results can be replicated in human beings, this herb could be used during radiation therapy as an additional, or adjunctive, treatment for the cancer itself, as well as for protection from radiation damage.

St. John's wort is an excellent antidepressant that also provides a remarkable range of other healing properties. Its ability to fight viruses is giving new hope to patients with diseases as varied as herpes and AIDS, while its wound-healing and antibacterial actions can offer protection against the multitude of potentially dangerous organisms in the world around us. Even better, its complex structure allows it to balance the immune system, helping to control inflammation as it boosts the body's ability to fight off disease. In the next chapter, I will explain how to use St. John's wort.

5

How to Use
St. John's Wort

At this point, you may be thinking, "St. John's wort sounds great. It can help me sleep better and it can lift my mood, all with minimal side effects. So how do I get started?" That's a good question, since, like many herbs, St. John's wort is available in any number of forms and dosages.

In this chapter, I will describe the various forms available, with their individual advantages and disadvantages. I'll also tell you about recommended dosages. As you will discover, the different products can contain varying quantities and concentrations of the active ingredients. In addition, there are differences in quality and potency. You also need to know about the occasional side effects, as well as the conditions under which you shouldn't take St. John's wort.

FORMS AND RECOMMENDED DOSAGE

There are many ways to take St. John's wort. The most common current form in North America is the capsule, containing dried extracts of the plant. On the other hand, European pharmaceutical manufacturers favor the use of tablets. Traditional tinctures have been used for centuries.

In the case of St. John's wort, some of its active ingredients have yet to be discovered. Still, we need a way of standardizing the product, that is, to have a consistent amount of product per dose. While the chemical hypericin was initially considered to be the main active ingredient of St. John's wort, current research indicates that it does not provide the major antidepressant activity. However, hypericin content is a convenient reference point when creating standardized extracts. You will find this on the label, with most products using a 0.3 percent concentration. This means that a 300-milligram (mg) capsule contains 0.9 mg of hypericin.

Extracts from as low as 0.125 percent up to 0.3 percent hypericin content have yielded positive results. The original studies used the lower concentration, while most current studies employ the 0.3 percent concentration. Be sure to use a standardized product that gives you a total of 1.0 to 2.7 mg of hypericin per day (equal to 300 to 900 mg of 0.3 percent hypericin).

The recommended daily dose will vary from individual to individual. One person may do well on 300 mg a day, while another may require 900 mg. Doses over 900 mg have been used, but I don't recommend using more than 1,200 mg, since it is not likely to increase the effect. The best dose is the lowest one that produces results for you.

Not all products utilize the same part of the herb. Some use only the unopened flowers, or buds. These contain the highest concentrations of active ingredients, so products made exclusively from buds are generally the most potent. The opened flowers of St. John's wort contain somewhat less hypericin, and the longer a flower has been open, the lower its hypericin level. This is likely to be true for the other active ingredients, as well. The next highest source of these plant chemicals is the leaf. The remainder of the plant, including the stalk and roots, is much lower in hypericin concentration. (See "Finding the Hypericin in St. John's Wort" on page 72.)

Because of these differing concentrations of active ingredients throughout the plant, products can vary widely. It is preferable to use products that are either all buds, or buds and flowers. Leaves tend to dilute the strength of the product, although a manufacturer can compensate for this by including more material in each capsule or tablet. Other factors include the growing and picking conditions—soil, season, even time of day.

Let's take a closer look at each form.

Capsules

Gelatin- or vegetable-based capsules filled with powdered dried herb is the most common form of administration in the United States. They come in a variety of strengths, so read the labels to ensure proper dosage.

Most capsules are in the 250 to 300 mg range of 0.3 percent hypericin. With lower-concentration capsules, you will need to take a higher dose—that is, more milligrams—for the same result. For people who need a lower dose, though, lower-concentration capsules may be just right.

Tablets

Tablets, which offer another option, consist of powdered herb compressed into a solid pill. Like capsules, tablets are more convenient than tinctures.

Finding the Hypericin in St. John's Wort

Not all parts of the St. John's wort plant have the same amount of hypericin and other active chemicals. Here are the amounts of hypericin by weight for various parts of the plant:

Flower petals	0.245%
Dried flowers	0.196% to 1.8%
Fresh flowers	0.09% to 0.12%
Whole plant with flower buds	0.042%
Whole plant with open flowers	0.036% to 0.2%
Young whole plant	0.027%
Stems	0.021%
Leaves	0.019%

Sources:
Benigni, R., Capra, C., and Cattorini, P.E. *Hypericum, Piante Medicinali: Chimica, Farmacologia e Terapia*. Milano: Inverni & Della Beffa, 1971.

Hänsel, R., Keller, K., Rimpler, H., and Schneider, G. *Hagers Handbuch der Pharmazeuischen Praxis*. Vol. 5. Berlin: Springer-Verlag, 1993.

Tinctures

Traditional herbalists prefer tinctures, which are liquid extracts produced by soaking the crushed herb in alcohol or glycerine. The oily, active ingredients in the herb seep out into the liquid. The remaining residue is then filtered out, resulting in a bright-red liquid that contains nearly all of the hypericin, pseudohypericin, and other active chemicals in the plant. Tinctures are normally available in brown glass bottles with medicine droppers attached to their caps.

The proper dosage depends on the severity of your condition, your body's own ability to absorb and utilize the tincture, and the product's potency.

When determining dosage, I tell my patients to start low, with a dropperful once or twice a day, and build up, adding one more after a few days, and so on, to a maximum of two dropperfuls two to three times daily. Unlike synthetic medicines, herbs have a lot of leeway between the effective dose and the excessive dose. It can be mixed with water or juice to disguise the taste.

To avoid the taste or effects (very minimal in this low concentration) of alcohol, leaving the tincture in warm water for few minutes will allow the alcohol to evaporate. I have found, though, that many people are reluctant to use tinctures because of the unusual taste, the difficulty in measuring, and the potential for spillage and breakage. Most of us in North America prefer our medicines in a premeasured, portable, odorless form. On the other hand, people like Ed Smith, renowned herbalist, say, "We were meant to taste what goes into our stomachs. The experience is part of the healing process."

TIPS FOR USING ST. JOHN'S WORT

It is essential to take some drugs on a set time schedule, such as once every four hours. This is because they are active in the body for only a short period of time, after which they are degraded by the liver and excreted. Fortunately, with St. John's wort, there is more flexibility. Studies have shown that two of the main chemicals in the herb, hypericin and pseudohypericin, have relatively long half-lives. A *half-life* is a scientific term that indicates the time it takes for one-half of the substance to be degraded in the body. Although the exact half-life depends on the dosage taken, studies show that hypericin and pseudohypericin have an average half-life of 25.8 hours and 25.0 hours, respectively. This means the herb is active twenty-four hours a day—working even while you sleep.

While it would be possible to take your entire daily dosage all at once, I do not recommend doing so, for several reasons. First, it is always preferable to give your body small doses of a substance on a frequent basis. This not only minimizes the potential for any side effects, but it permits a more steady concentration of the active chemicals in your blood and brain. This consideration can be particularly important when you first start using the herb. Second, the antidepressant benefits of St. John's wort may be enhanced by herbal components other than hypericin and pseudohypericin, and these could have shorter half-lives. Thus, more frequent doses may in fact be necessary to receive full advantage from the herb.

I recommend taking St. John's wort with breakfast, lunch, and dinner. Taking it with food reduces its concentration, minimizing any possible nausea or gastrointestinal upset (see page 84). Taking the herb with meals also makes it easier to incorporate into your daily routine. On the other hand, if convenience is important, it is fine to take two doses in the morning and one with dinner.

It can take as long as six weeks for the antidepressant effects of St. John's wort to begin. Once the effect stabilizes, you can stay on the herb as long as necessary. It's a good idea to try tapering off after a few months, but this requires close observation, to ensure that you don't inadvertently slip back into depression. Why "inadvertently?" Because sometimes the patient is the last to notice this slippage. In fact, family members or close friends are often better observers, so it is useful to enroll them in the process. I have also had patients early in treatment—on either natural or synthetic medication—tell me that they haven't noticed positive changes, while family members have noticed marked improvements.

There are individuals who self-monitor very well. They will start taking St. John's wort again as soon as they feel they are slipping, and often find that the benefits kick in faster than when they first started using the herb. Perhaps the brain is somehow "trained" in its response, or perhaps there is a residual level of St. John's wort in the body.

Carmen is a good example of someone who self-monitors her use of St. John's wort.

A 38-year-old divorced mother of two teenaged daughters, Carmen started taking St. John's wort after hearing how it helped a friend through a difficult period and continued to help her afterwards. Carmen "began to take St. John's wort tincture, three droppers a day, sometimes four. I noticed a change almost immediately. I also take extra on days that I'm particularly stressed, and it helps put things in perspective. I work as a travel agent, and it gets intense at times.

"Also, living with teenagers can be trying. I found myself yelling at them a lot—I would just say what came to mind, and be sorry afterward, till the next time. However, soon after starting the St. John's wort, I was in the shower and noticed that my 15-year-old had taken my shampoo for the umpteenth time. Dripping wet, I put on a towel, and went to retrieve the shampoo. Rather than running out raving at my

daughter, I was calm." Carmen found, like many others
who take St. John's wort, that she could deal with such
situations in a kinder, more understanding fashion, de-
spite being upset. "Our relationship then began to im-
prove. We communicated better."

She also noticed that PMS and menstrual cramps,
from which she had suffered for most of her life, had
disappeared. "I have told lots of my friends about St.
John's wort, and they are also doing great."

OTHER HERBS AND COMBINATION PRODUCTS

St. John's wort works well in combination with a number of other herbs and natural remedies. Individual
herbs are made up of many compounds that function
together as a healing unit, the whole being greater than
the sum of its parts. By the same token, various herbs
can work together with a synergy that enhances and re-
inforces the positive effects of each. Herbal effects tend
to ripple throughout the body, strengthening and supporting many organs at once. While there are certain
herbs that should not be used together, such combinations are infrequent, and far less likely to cause harm
than many drug combinations.

Professional herbalists and natural health practitioners
have formulated numerous combination products with
St. John's wort. A number of these products are com-
mercially available. They draw upon centuries of herbal
tradition as well as current research. Of course, since
we are all different in our biochemical makeup, common sense should always be exercised in taking any
product, even a natural one. If you are unsure of
whether or not you should use a particular product or
herb, consult an herbalist or other wholistic health care
practitioner.

Individual herbalists use different combinations to

fight depression and related disorders. David Winston, a founding member of the American Herbalists Guild, believes in using the right formula for each type of depression. For example, in treating depression related to PMS and menopause, he recommends St. John's wort in combination with blue vervain and motherwort, with the addition of black cohosh to combat "sudden black cloud" feelings. For decreased libido, he uses damiana. For SAD, Winston recommends lemon balm in combination with St. John's wort. Terry Willard, director of Wild Rose College of Natural Healing, recommends a combination of St. John's wort, Reishi mushroom, and kava (see below) for anxiety.

Some of the more common and effective St. John's wort combinations use kava, ginseng, schizandra, and ginkgo biloba. There are also women's tonics and insomnia formulations.

Kava

Kava-kava (often just called "kava"), the root of the *Piper methysticum* plant, is an excellent partner for St. John's wort, especially for those individuals with mixed anxiety and depression. Used for centuries in the South Pacific, kava promotes mental and physical relaxation while reducing muscle tension, without causing the drowsiness associated with tranquilizers such as Valium and Xanax. Research has shown it to actually enhance alertness and concentration. The rapid response of kava will provide needed relief during the several weeks it may take for St. John's wort to have an effect. The usual dose of kava for anxiety and tension is 100 mg of 70 percent standardized kavalactones (the kava equivalent of hypericin), three times a day. For insomnia, the dose is 200 to 300 mg before bed. A German study found it to be successful in treating

the depression, anxiety, and insomnia related to menopause.

There are formulas that combine St. John's wort and
kava with vitamins B_6 and B_{12}, important cofactors in
the treatment of depression. Some even add the amino
acid tyrosine, another natural antidepressant. (For more
information on the nutritional approach to depression relief, see Chapter 8.)

I find kava combinations particularly useful in older
individuals, such as Harry.

> Harry, a 76-year-old man with a history of prostate can-
> cer and chronic constipation, was brought into my of-
> fice by his wife, Molly. "If I could buy a separate house,
> I would," she said. "He's impossible: depressed, nega-
> tive, cranky, and tired, and he can't sleep. Either give
> him something for his mood, or give me something to
> put me out of my misery!"
>
> Most conventional doctors would strongly consider
> an antidepressant and possibly a sleeping pill, although
> the side effects could aggravate Harry's medical prob-
> lems. Instead, I prescribed a variety of natural prod-
> ucts: kava for anxiety; the amino acid tyrosine, a
> natural antidepressant; ginseng for adrenal support;
> and a combination of valerian, passion flower, and
> skullcap for sleep. In addition, I added 300 milligrams
> of St. John's wort twice daily. The combination
> worked. In three weeks, Harry was "his old self," ac-
> cording to a grateful Molly.

Older patients such as Harry often react poorly to
medication because their livers cannot process synthetic
substances as effectively as they could when they were
younger. In fact, older people quite often need nutritional supplements to replenish and support other systems, as well.

Ginseng

A formula that is particularly good for stress combines St. John's wort with Siberian ginseng (*Eleutherococcus senticosus*). Ginseng is an adaptogen, which means it acts to regulate and balance the system. In particular, it supports and replenishes the adrenal glands, an essential part of our stress-fighting system that often become depleted in those suffering from anxiety and depression (see Chapter 3).

George is a good example of how a combination treatment can really make a difference.

George, a 30-year-old magazine journalist, had recently been through a divorce. He was depressed and having more than his usual share of colds. George had no desire to go to work, even though he had always loved his job, and felt too tired even to exercise, though he had always been a self-described "exercise nut." Weekly psychotherapy helped him to understand why he was depressed, but was of minimal help. His naturopath suggested that he take 300 milligrams of St. John's wort two to three times a day, along with Siberian ginseng. In three weeks, he was not only his old self, but even better! George stayed on the combination for several months before stopping it gradually. Whenever he felt stressed, he would resume taking the herbs for a while.

It is likely that George had always been mildly depressed without realizing it, and that his divorce aggravated the depression. Note that he could resume taking the herbs with immediate benefits when he needed them, unlike synthetic antidepressants, which can take several weeks to produce positive results if resumed.

Schizandra

Schizandra (*Schizandra chinensis*), like ginseng, helps the body resist the effects of stress. It also protects and supports the liver, the major detoxification center of the body, and acts as an antioxidant. Furthermore, schizandra appears to have a calming effect on the brain. Dr. Dan Beilin, a natural health practitioner, developed a formula that combines it with St. John's wort, kava, orchid extract, zinc salts, and several other herbs to produce a mood-balancing formula.

Ginkgo Biloba

One of the best-researched herbs in Europe, ginkgo is also one of the oldest. It is used widely in Europe, and increasingly in North America, to increase blood supply to the brain and improve mental functioning. Gingko appears to have a pronounced antidepressant action, possibly due to a serotonin-enhancing effect (see Chapter 3). In one study, both old and young rats were treated with ginkgo. The older rats showed a 33 percent increase in serotonin receptor binding sites, despite the fact that they had fewer receptors to begin with. In other studies, ginkgo has been shown to be an effective antidepressant when compared with a placebo. It has few side effects, and they are mild. The dosage is 24 percent ginkgo flavonglycosides (the ginkgo equivalent of hypericin), 40 to 80 mg, two to three times a day. A response occurs in anywhere from two to twelve weeks.

I have seen elderly patients who appeared withdrawn and barely functioning come out of their shells and interact normally after a few weeks of ginkgo treatment. These gains are lost if the program is not maintained, and return when the ginkgo is resumed.

Women's Tonics

Hormonal support formulas for women, including the herbs dong quai, vitex, and black cohosh, can provide welcome relief from the symptoms of PMS, menstrual cramps, and menopause. As mentioned earlier, St. John's wort is an excellent treatment for such conditions, and these added herbs serve to enhance its effects.

Bill Brevoort of the East Earth Herb Company says that the heart and mind are the same character in Chinese medicine. When given for depression, St. John's wort stimulates the circulation of heart energy. In turn, the heart needs to be supported and replenished with an herb such as dong quai. A particularly useful herb, dong quai is also an adaptogen, immune stimulant, liver and lung tonic, and regulator of estrogen effects.

Insomnia

As I've said before, herbal sleeping aids are greatly preferable to pharmaceuticals, since they do not produce habituation or addiction. There is no withdrawal, no interference with REM or dream sleep, and no morning hangover effect. Some useful herbs, generally available in combinations, are: valerian (150 to 300 mg of 0.8 percent valeric acid), hops, passion flower, and skullcap. As noted, both St. John's wort and kava have a sleep-regulating effect.

You may wonder why I have not suggested the hormone melatonin. I believe it is overused as a sleeping agent. The best use seems to be in small doses (1 to 2 mg) at bedtime for coping with jet lag or adjusting to shift work. In the elderly, it can also be useful when a lack of the hormone is evident. It appears that St. John's wort may have its own melatonin-enhancing effect, allowing a more natural production and release of this hormone. One study by Demisch and colleagues showed that

St. John's wort, taken at the rate of ninety drops of tincture every day over a three-week period, significantly increased nighttime melatonin levels.

WHERE YOU CAN BUY ST. JOHN'S WORT

St. John's wort is available in most health food stores, pharmacies, and—with its new popularity—many other stores as well. In the United States, herbs taken for medicinal purposes fall, like pharmaceuticals, under the aegis of the Food and Drug Administration (FDA). Most recently, their use has been controlled by the 1994 Dietary Supplement Health and Education Act (DSHEA), which allows certain claims to be made regarding an herb's effects on the "structure and function" of the body, as long as it already has been declared safe. This was a hard-won compromise that only came about due to persistent lobbying by thousands of citizens, supplement suppliers, and health practitioners.

In Canada, there are provisions for herbs to be designated as "folklore medicines" under the Health Protection Branch, which is part of the National Health and Welfare Department. Labeling can both inform the consumer of an herb's therapeutic use and regulate the dosage. There are still restrictions regarding use of herbs, and a number of products available in the United States are banned in Canada. Fortunately, St. John's wort is not on the banned list. (See Appendix D.)

You will need to choose among various brands, strengths, and forms of St. John's wort. Be sure to pick a brand that is standardized, because this will ensure the same quantity of active ingredients in each dose. Even so, there are differences in quality between brands. Some people have reported doing well on St. John's wort until they changed brands, despite a label showing an equivalent strength. They found that the effect was simply not the same. Upon resuming use of the former brand, their symptoms improved once again. Conversely, apparent failures of St. John's wort for some individuals became great successes when they switched brands. Prices can also vary widely for similar products, so do some comparison shopping. I prefer using a trusted source, even if the material costs more, although price does not necessarily reflect quality. Some inexpensive brands are excellent.

Other sources for St. John's wort include the in-house supplies of physicians, naturopaths, and other natural health practitioners. For my own office, I choose supplements from a variety of manufacturers, always looking for the best quality at the lowest price. You can also order St. John's wort by mail (see Appendix B for a list of suppliers).

Look for brands that are certified organic, meaning they are free of pesticides and other synthetic chemicals. Organic herbs often have higher nutrient concentrations as well, yielding more healing power per flower. Wildcrafted herbs, picked and processed fresh from the woods and meadows where they grow, are an excellent choice. A friend of mine who owns an herb company in southern Oregon told me that during a recent spike in demand for St. John's wort, he could scarcely keep up with orders. He hired high school students on summer vacation to pick huge bags of the wild herb, which grows quite abundantly in his area. The students made money, and the company was able to fill its orders.

Warning: This same friend says you must know your territory before picking wild roadside St. John's wort, which may have been sprayed with herbicides by cattle ranchers or highway maintenance crews. This can lead to a serious toxic reaction.

OCCASIONAL SIDE EFFECTS

St. John's wort is remarkably safe. Compared with Prozac and the other prescription antidepressants, it has a very low incidence of side effects. This makes it the antidepressant of choice for older people, who are more likely to experience side effects from synthetic medications. Moreover, even when these side effects do occur, they tend to be milder than those produced by the manufactured drugs and generally disappear at a lower dosage, while maintaining the antidepressant effect. In any case, all side effects stop as soon as the intake stops. St. John's wort does not have adverse effects when mixed with alcohol. In addition, it is not addictive, nor does it produce withdrawal symptoms when you stop taking it. The *habituation* that commonly occurs with synthetic drugs—that is, the need for a higher dosage to maintain the effect—does not occur with the herb. All this gives St. John's wort a clear advantage over the other available medications.

In Chapter 4, I briefly mentioned a German drug monitoring study. Out of the 3,250 persons participating in this controlled experiment by Woelk, Burkard, and Gruenwald, only 79—or 2.4 percent—of them reported side effects. These included gastrointestinal symptoms (0.55 percent), allergic reactions (0.2 percent), anxiety (0.26 percent), and dizziness (0.15 percent). Moreover, 1.5 percent found the side effects so intense that they had to discontinue therapy. Comparable studies on prescription drugs have found side-effect frequencies and discontinuation rates as much as ten times higher! Let's take a closer look at these side effects:

- *Gastrointestinal symptoms.* This is the most common side effect reported by users and includes nausea, loss of appetite, and abdominal pains. If you experience gastrointestinal symptoms, which can occur with any substance (even a placebo), simply take your dose with a meal.

- *Allergic reactions.* This includes skin rashes and itching.

- *Phototoxicity.* In the past, phototoxicity, or severe sunburn, was a major concern because light-haired cattle and sheep, after consuming great quantities of the plant while grazing in the sun, developed serious sunburns. This led the Food and Drug Administration (FDA) to put St. John's wort on its unsafe list, where it remained for many years. However, a 1993 human study found that the usual therapeutic doses used in depression are so small that the probability of phototoxicity is very low. The only people who are likely to experience phototoxicity are persons with AIDS who are taking extremely high amounts of the herb for its antiviral properties. To be cautious, fair-skinned individuals taking high doses should use sunscreen and avoid major sun exposure.

- *Anxiety.* A few St. John's wort users report this side effect. Users of the selective serotonin uptake re-uptake inhibitors (SSRIs), such as Prozac, report a far higher rate (9 percent) of anxiety, particularly at the start of the treatment program. This anxiety should disappear after the first few weeks. The best course of action is to call your doctor and reduce the dosage until the anxiety resolves itself. I have heard of individuals who developed increased irritability on St. John's wort, which disappeared upon stopping the herb. We are all different, so we can be affected in different ways. It's important to be a good observer, to trust your experience, and to act accordingly.

PRECAUTIONS AND CONTRAINDICATIONS

The depression studies to date have dealt with adults only, and with no medical condition other than their depression. The jury is still out on how St. John's wort can affect other groups.

If you are over age sixty-five, have a medical condition, or are taking any medication, be sure to speak with your doctor before starting to use St. John's wort. While the herb is much safer than the prescription antidepressants, these factors may make you more sensitive to its effects, and you may need a lower dosage. This is especially true if you have a liver or kidney disease. Since these two organs are involved in the processing of all medications, the concentrations of the herb's active chemicals can become excessive, even toxic.

While there is no evidence that St. John's wort can produce birth defects, I advise pregnant and nursing women not to use it until more research is available. It is recommended that children under twelve should also not be given St. John's wort, since we have no specific research in this area. Of course, children, some quite young, are given a variety of antidepressants, and common sense would say that St. John's wort would be a safer substitute. In Europe, St. John's wort is a common treatment for bedwetting in children. But until more data is available, it should be administered with care under appropriate medical supervision.

It was initially recommended that those taking St. John's wort should avoid foods containing the amino acid tyramine, as well as MAO-inhibiting drugs such as 5-hydroxytryptophan and L-dopa, for fear of causing an unsafe rise in blood pressure. However, hundreds of thousands of people with high blood pressure in Germany use St. John's wort without any problems. Newer research has shown that the MAO effect seems to occur only in test tubes, *not* in people. In fact, St. John's wort likely works through other mechanisms, such as inhibiting the uptake of serotonin into the neurons (Chapter 3).

USING ST. JOHN'S WORT
WITH OTHER ANTIDEPRESSANTS

I have used St. John's wort with patients who were already on antidepressants, including Prozac, Zoloft, Effexor (venlafaxine hydrochloride), and the tricyclics (see Chapter 7), as well as those taking such amino acids as tryptophan. Of possible concern in these cases is "serotonin syndrome," or an excessive serotonin buildup in the brain. There is no record of this occurring, despite thousands of people having taken the combination of St. John's wort and SSRIs. When asked about this possibility, Dr. Jerry Cott, a psychopharmacologist at the National Institute of Mental Health, asserted that "there have been no deaths or toxic reactions, no adverse interactions related to MAO inhibition, and no incidents of serotonin syndrome reported in the literature. There is no clear evidence in . . . animal studies or in human trials that serotonin is even potentiated by St. John's wort." What is clear is that more research work is needed before we fully understand how this herb works.

One of the the most common questions I am asked concerns the best way to switch from an antidepressant to St. John's wort. There is no research data on this subject, only the experiences of many patients and their physicians.We all look forward to having definitive reports in the future. For now, I can say that the process must be done under a doctor's supervision, preferably the one who prescribed the antidepressant. If your doctor is reluctant to do this, I would encourage you to share this book with him or her. The doctor can thus become familiar with the clinical use of St. John's wort. He or she can also look up the research evidence in Chapter 6, including an explanation of why there is so little North American research on this subject. Appendix C will provide your doctor with the appropriate changeover protocol.

It is important to point out that switching from a synthetic antidepressant to St. John's wort without appropriate supervision can pose serious problems. For example, if the antidepressant is stopped abruptly, a rebound effect could result, leading to renewed anxiety and depression. Or, if St. John's wort is combined with the wrong drug, there can be negative consequences. This is especially true of MAO-inhibiting antidepressants such as Nardil (phenelzine sulfate) or Parnate (tranylcypromine sulfate). (See Appendix C.) Also, as we have discussed, St. John's wort is not recommended as the sole treatment in major depression, and its use in bipolar disorder remains a question.

As we've seen in this chapter, St. John's wort is pretty simple to use—just take it with meals. While the side effects are generally minimal, it is *essential* to speak with your doctor if you have a preexisting medical condition or if you are already taking an antidepressant. Finding a doctor open to natural therapies may be an important consideration—see Appendix B and read "How to Find an Understanding Doctor" on page 141. In the next chapter, I'll discuss the studies that support the use of St. John's wort.

6

Depression and St. John's Wort— Looking at the Proof

S t. John's wort has been used successfully for thousands of years. People all around the world, from the ancient Greeks to the Native Americans, found this herb to be a powerful remedy for a variety of problems, from depression to serious wounds (see Chapter 4).

In this chapter, after first providing some basic information on research studies in general, I'll discuss the studies that have been done on St. John's wort. The results speak for themselves.

WHAT YOU NEED TO KNOW ABOUT RESEARCH STUDIES

Research studies are the backbone of conventional medicine. They have provided us with a wealth of valuable information in all fields, including human biology and the health sciences. As useful as studies are, however, they do have their shortcomings, especially when they focus on an area as subtle and complex as the mind-body connection. In addition, the whole issue of research and health is complicated by factors that determine which therapies receive funding and which do not.

The Science of Studies

Historical knowledge, the foundation for many of the modern herbal texts, has served as sufficient proof of an herb's effectiveness. Modern science, however, has developed a rigorous system of standards in an effort to ensure that bias and preconceived notions are not misinterpreted as scientific fact. Scientists develop a *hypothesis*, essentially an educated guess about a specific set of facts, and then test it under controlled conditions.

In drug tests, this often involves comparing effects experienced by people who take the test substance with those experienced by people who take an identical-looking but inert substance known as a *placebo*, or "sugar pill." In other tests, two different test substances are compared with each other. Usually these studies are *double-blind*, meaning that neither the researchers nor the study participants are aware of who is taking which product. The results of these experiments are then submitted to scientific journals for publication, subject to the approval of a committee of respected scientists in the field.

With due respect to the scientific method, there may be a basic fallacy in the desire to control for the *placebo effect*. This effect refers to the feelings or responses reported by someone taking a placebo, and is based on an expectation of results. In other words, if you think the pill will help you, it may very well do so. Conversely, if you think you'll have side effects, that may also happen. A placebo is not "nothing" or "just a sugar pill." The innate ability of the body to heal itself is awesome, and what we know as the placebo effect is actually an example of how the mind affects the body. Just think about it: After surgery, for example, is it the sutures holding the wound together that does the healing? Or, after a fracture, is it the cast that repairs the break? Not at all. It is the wisdom of the body. By the same token, the placebo response is always present. It is the innate intelligence of the mind-body connection, the inner healer. Without it, wounds would stay open, bacteria would cause overwhelming infection, and fractures would not heal. We know that hypnosis can accelerate both emotional and physical healing. The answer to the "mind-over-matter" question is that "mind *is* matter."

Here is an excellent example. An experiment was performed in which two groups of patients were given a painkilling substance. The placebo group did almost as well as the treatment group, with positive expectation underlying the result. Then the placebo group was given a shot of naloxone—and the good effects of the medication were reversed! What happened? Naloxone is a known "opiate antagonist," a substance that blocks the effects of painkilling chemicals. In this case, the naloxone blocked endorphins produced by the patients' own bodies, and the placebo response was stopped. The conclusion we should reach from this experiment is that the placebo effect is a real, measurable product of the body's biochemistry. We can also conclude that a healing substance, whether synthetic or natural, will be utilized more effectively by an individual who has a positive attitude and faith in its efficacy.

Doctors, Studies, and Drug Companies

When patients ask about herbs or other natural remedies, most conventional doctors say, "But there's no proof." Why? In most cases, doctors simply don't know about natural therapies. Drug companies are their main source of new information, and most natural products do not have a major corporation behind them. In Europe—where herbs are classified with other pharmaceutical products, prescribed by doctors, and covered by national health plans—it's a different story.

Research is costly, running into the millions. Because herbal medicine is accepted in Europe as a legitimate form of therapy, European drug companies have the financial incentive to do the necessary research. In North America, this is not the case. Here, pharmaceutical companies will bear the cost of research only if they can patent the new products that result from it. The worldwide antidepressant market, for example, is worth an estimated $6 billion annually. Natural products such as herbs can't be patented, and discoveries made about them become public domain. Therefore, the companies will not put money into studying them, since there would be an insufficient return on their investment.

As a result of the drug companies' huge investment in their products, and of their collaboration with medical schools for research purposes, much of the information taught to doctors in medical school and beyond comes from the companies themselves. Most doctors are trained in *allopathic medicine*, that is, the conventional drug-and-surgery approach, with relatively few going on to practice *alternative* or *wholistic medicine*, which taps into the body's own healing powers.

However, demand is growing in North America for a more natural approach to medicine, including the use of such products such as herbs. Therefore, it is likely that the American pharmaceutical industry will follow the European lead, creating refined extracts so they can patent their products. Unfortunately, this involves focusing on the so-called "active" ingredient(s) and removing the "extra material" that actually make herbs the powerful healers they are.

SUZUKI AND COLLEAGUES: THE PIONEER STUDY

One of the earliest studies on St. John's wort, now a classic, was by Suzuki and colleagues. In 1984, this team studied the effects on monoamine oxidase (MAO) of hypericin, which was thought at the time to be the herb's active ingredient. As you may recall from Chapter 3, MAO is an enzyme that reduces the amount of neurotransmitters in the synapses between the nerve cells. This leads to an increase in neurotransmitter levels and a decrease in depressive feelings. Suzuki's team did this study *in vitro*, which means "in a test tube," as opposed to *in vivo*, which means in a living subject. They found that there was a direct correlation between the concentration of hypericin and the amount of MAO inhibition.

This study led doctors to believe that St. John's wort's antidepressive action was mainly achieved through MAO inhibition, which in turn led to specific food restrictions associated with the herb (see page 103). Also, since hypericin was considered the plant's primary antidepressant ingredient, this study led to the current practice of referring to the hypericin content when creating standardized extracts. More recent research has found other aspects of the plant to be more active in this regard. However, there is no question that Suzuki's team provided a major impetus for research into the medicinal value of St. John's wort.

MORE STUDIES PROVIDE MORE PROOF

This has been a very fruitful period for St. John's wort research. A large number of controlled studies have come from Germany, where *Hypericum perforatum* has been an accepted part of the psychiatrist's medicine bag for decades.

Now, there is mainstream interest in the United States

in St. John's wort. The National Institute of Mental Health, a division of the National Institutes of Health (NIH), is about to embark on a series of studies aimed at evaluating the efficacy and safety of a standardized hypericum extract in treating depression. This research, which will be conducted at numerous locations, will be done in collaboration with the Office of Alternative Medicine and the NIH Office of Dietary Supplements.

Two landmark publications heralded the widespread interest in St. John's wort throughout the English-speaking world. In 1994, the *Journal of Geriatric Psychiatry and Neurology*, edited by Michael Jenike of the Harvard Medical School, dedicated the entire October issue to hypericum. "Hypericum: A Novel Antidepressant" looked at sixteen studies that supported the use of the herb in fighting depression.

Then, in 1996, a significant and extensive review article was published in the *British Medical Journal*. The authors did a *meta-analysis*, or comparison, of twenty-three randomized clinical trials to see what overall conclusions they could reach. Fifteen studies compared the herb with a placebo, and eight compared it with conventional antidepressants, covering a total of 1,757 patients.

The four- to eight-week placebo studies, performed in the private practices of various psychiatrists, internists, and general practitioners, found St. John's wort to be significantly superior. The daily dosage levels ranged from 350 mg to 1,000 mg of standardized hypericum extract, or 0.4 mg to 2.7 mg per day of hypericin. An average of 55.1 percent of the hypericum users responded to the treatment, much higher than the 22.3 percent response rate of the placebo group.

In both groups, individual depression levels were measured according to the Hamilton Depression Scale (HAMD), a widely accepted diagnostic tool. The examiner assigns a numerical value to each of a variety of depressive symptoms, such as feelings of fear or sadness, sleep disturbance, or impaired concentration. These are then added up to give a total score. The higher the number, the more intense the depression. The HAMD scores of the groups taking St. John's wort were 4.4 points lower at the end of the study than the scores of those taking the placebo, indicating a greater improvement.

Only 0.4 percent of the persons taking St. John's wort dropped out because of side effects, as compared with *1.6 percent among placebo users.* As I mentioned before, the placebo effect is a powerful one.

This meta-analysis also compared the herb with a number of antidepressant drugs, including maprotiline hydrochloride (Ludiomil), imipramine hydrochloride (Tofranil), bromazepam (a drug similar to Valium), amitriptyline hydrochloride (Elavil), and desipramine hydrochloride (Norpramin; see Chapter 7 for information on the synthetic antidepressants). Extract dosages ranged from 500 mg to 900 mg daily. These studies showed that St. John's wort did slightly better than the antidepressants in eliciting a positive response, 63.9 percent versus 58.5 percent. In addition, only 0.8 percent of people taking the herb dropped out of the study because of side effects, while 3.0 percent of those on drug treatment ended their participation early.

The studies that appeared in both the *Journal of Geriatric Psychiatry and Neurology* and the *British Medical Journal* were done in Germany. German research standards are considered high enough that the results of these studies are reliable. We will look at four representative studies.

Harrer and Sommer (1994) looked at St. John's wort's ability to treat mild to moderate depression. In this four-week, double-blind study, 105 outpatients were given either 300 mg of 0.3 percent St. John's wort extract or a placebo, three times per day.

Both groups started out with nearly identical HAMD scores. Yet after only two weeks, the average HAMD score of the group taking the herb dropped from 15.81 to 9.64, and two weeks later, to 7.17. The placebo group, on the other hand, dropped from 15.83 to 12.28 by the second week, and to 11.30 by the fourth week. All in all, 67 percent of the active group had HAMD scores that showed a response to treatment, while only 28 percent of the placebo group responded. This means that two-thirds of the people using St. John's wort had a significant reduction in their depressive symptoms in only four weeks. Additionally, there were no reported side effects.

Among the St. John's wort users, there were particularly impressive improvements in the symptoms of depression, such as feelings of sadness, hopelessness, helplessness, and uselessness, in addition to reductions in insomnia, fear, headache, cardiac symptoms, and exhaustion.

A double-blind study, by Hänsgen and colleagues, reached the same conclusions. Seventy-two depressed patients received either a 300 mg tablet of St. John's wort extract or a placebo three times a day. The patients, aged eighteen to seventy years, met the criteria for major depression but were not psychotic or suicidal. The individuals had been depressed from a minimum of two weeks to a maximum of six months. After four weeks, all the study participants took St. John's wort for an additional two weeks. This procedure, called a *crossover*, allowed the researchers to see what would happen to the hypericum users when they continued treatment for fourteen more days, while letting the scientists measure the response of the former placebo group to a short trial of St. John's wort.

Despite the fact that the active group started with an average HAMD score slightly higher than the control group (21.2 versus 20.4), those persons taking the herbal extract experienced substantially greater reductions in their depressive symptoms during the first four weeks. The HAMD scores of the St. John's wort users dropped to 9.2, while the average score of the placebo group declined to only 14.7.

During the fifth and sixth weeks, the hypericum users continued to improve. Their average HAMD score fell another 32 percent to 6.3, for a total drop of 70 percent in six weeks. Those who switched from the placebo to St. John's wort for the last two weeks experienced reductions similar to those of the extract users. Only three patients reported mild side effects, and two of these were actually using the placebo!

Harrer and colleagues (1994) compared St. John's wort with a synthetic antidepressant called maprotiline. The four-week, double-blind study looked at a group of 102 patients. Each received the usually recommended amounts of St. John's wort or maprotiline hydrochloride. The researchers found that the two products had equivalent effectiveness. HAMD scores for the hypericum users dropped by 49 percent compared with a 51 percent reduction for maprotiline. However, St. John's wort produced 43 percent fewer side effects than the synthetic drug.

Vorbach and colleagues (1994) compared St. John's wort with imipramine hydrochloride. In this randomized, double-blind study, the researchers divided 135 depressed patients into two groups. Each group received the usually recommended dosages of the two products for six weeks. Despite the fact that the St. John's wort group started with a slightly higher HAMD score, patients using the herb had a better response to treatment. Their scores dropped by 56 percent, from 20.2 to 8.8, while those of the imipramine users declined 45 percent, from 19.4 to 10.7.

The St. John's wort group also had greater improvements in the severity of their illnesses, according to the Clinical Global Impressions (CGI) scale, another measure of depression. Nearly 82 percent of patients on the herb were classified as having improved, compared with only 63 percent of those using imipramine. None of those taking St. John's wort reported a worsening in their condition, whereas two patients on imipramine became more depressed. Despite the greater effectiveness of St. John's wort, it had half as many side effects, with all but one case being mild. Patients using imipramine indicated that a third of their side effects were either moderate or severe.

SEASONAL AFFECTIVE DISORDER

This powerful herb is also helpful in the treatment of seasonal affective disorder. As noted in Chapter 4, people with SAD suffer depressive symptoms in the autumn and winter months due to a lack of light exposure, which can trigger hormonal changes in the brain. Symptoms include fatigue, depressed mood, anxiety, reduced activity, increased appetite and sleep requirements, and reduced libido. Light therapy has become the standard treatment. It now appears that St. John's wort is effective, as well.

To determine the effectiveness of St. John's wort in treating SAD, Martinez and colleagues studied twenty patients aged twenty-nine to sixty-three with initial HAMD scores of at least 20. The test subjects were divided into two groups. One group received standard light therapy (3,000 lux for two hours each day) while the other group was treated with dim light (less than 300 lux for the same time period). Both groups were given 900 mg of herbal extract per day (equal to 2.7 mg of hypericin daily). The researchers then measured the changes in HAMD scores during the four-week experiment.

The group that received bright light showed a 72 percent drop in their average HAMD score (to 6.1), while the group treated with dim light had a drop of 60 percent (to 8.2). Therefore, the researchers concluded that St. John's wort is almost as effective as light therapy, although the combination of hypericum and light therapy is still likely to be superior. St. John's wort can offer more convenient relief to persons with SAD, making the need for light therapy not as critical.

These and other studies reflect St. John's wort's effectiveness in the treatment of mild to moderate depression and seasonal affective disorder. Research continues on this valuable herb, including trials in the United States. In the next chapter, I'll discuss the synthetic antidepressants.

7

Prozac and Beyond—
The Synthetic Antidepressants

Beginning in the 1950s, scientists developed a number of synthetic drugs for the treatment of depression, which represented a major step forward at the time. Prior to these discoveries, conventional psychiatrists were limited to psychotherapy, able only to listen and talk to their patients, trying to clarify and resolve the underlying psychological factors of depression. While these methods remain vital parts of psychiatric treatment, the invention of new drugs ushered in a promising new era.

There are three principal types of antidepressant medications: the tricyclic drugs, the monoamine oxidase inhibitors (MAOIs), and the selective serotonin re-uptake inhibitors (SSRIs). There are also three drugs that are chemically distinct from these types and each other: Wellbutrin, Desyrel, and Effexor. Classes differ in their mechanisms of action and side effects. However, they all have several things in common. They are effective in reducing depressive symptoms in 60 to 80 percent of the persons who use them. They also take from a month to six weeks to produce their full effects, although there can be side effects and changes in mood can occur much sooner.

In this chapter, I'll discuss the different classes of drugs before taking a closer look at the issue of side effects.

THE TRICYCLICS

The tricyclic drugs were the first antidepressant medications. They dominated the market for more than twenty years, and are still used today, though less frequently. They work by desensitizing a receptor in the neuron that absorbs the neurotransmitters norepinephrine and dopamine into the cells. This results in higher levels of these two chemicals in the synapse, and consequent improvements in mood. (See Chapter 3.)

The first one in this category was imipramine hydrochloride (Tofranil). More recent additions to this group include amitriptyline hydrochloride (Elavil, Limbitrol, Endep), desipramine hydrochloride (Norpramin), doxepin hydrochloride (Adapin, Sinequan), nortriptyline hydrochloride (Pamelor, Aventyl), and protriptyline hydrochloride (Vivactil).

A serious problem with the tricyclics is their level of side effects, particularly in patients over age sixty-five. They interfere with the body's control of blood pressure, which can lead to dizziness and even fainting spells. The drowsiness they produce makes it hazardous to drive. Some patients experience arrhythmias, or irregularities in heartbeat, as well. Additional side effects include sedation, dry mouth, blurred vision, confusion, weight gain, flulike symptoms, sweating, rashes, nausea, constipation or diarrhea, difficulty with urination, impotence or impaired erection in men, inhibited orgasm in women, nightmares, and anxiety.

Due to these effects, tricyclics are not usually prescribed, except when cost is a consideration, since they are considerably cheaper than the SSRIs. Because the tricyclics are an older class of drug, their patents have already run out, and the generic brands are more competitively priced. Some doctors will prescribe either doxepin or desipramine to be taken at bedtime in order to counter the insomnia that often occurs with Prozac.

THE MONOAMINE OXIDASE INHIBITORS

The monoamine oxidase inhibitors, or MAOIs, have a different mechanism of action than the other antidepressants. They work by reducing the quantity of the enzyme MAO within the synapse. The function of the enzyme is to help transport neurotransmitters, particularly norepinephrine, into the neurons. When MAO is inhibited, there is a greater supply of neurotransmitters in the synapse. This usually results in a reduction of depressive symptoms. The MAOIs seem to be particularly effective for atypical depression, in which depression is accompanied by oversleeping, overeating, and anxiety. This class of antidepressant includes phenelzine sulfate (Nardil) and tranylcypromine sulfate (Parnate).

While the MAOIs have fewer side effects than the tricyclic drugs, they can still cause problems in some individuals. Some common side effects include insomnia, impotence and other sexual dysfunction, dizziness, weight gain, and water retention. They can also produce a dangerous elevation in blood pressure, if the patient consumes substances containing the amino acid tyramine. These foods include all cheeses except cottage cheese and cream cheese, all forms of alcohol, pickled or smoked meats or fish, liver, sausage, salami, yeast, and fava beans. Persons taking MAOIs also need to watch their consumption of yogurt, sour cream, tomatoes, spinach, eggplant, avocado, soy sauce, raisins, plums, and bananas. Certain over-the-counter remedies, such as decongestants and antihistamines, must also be avoided. Needless to say, these restrictions put a crimp in most people's diets, so psychiatrists are less likely to prescribe them.

Because it was originally believed that St. John's wort worked through MAO inhibition (see Chapter 6), current sources on the herb still list the MAOI food restrictions. However, it is now quite clear that St. John's wort is not likely to have this effect, making the warnings unnecessary.

If the MAOIs and SSRIs are combined, there is the potential for a dangerous reaction known as the "serotonin syndrome" (see Chapter 5). Therefore, it is essential that there be at least a two-week period when switching from a MAOI to a SSRI, and a five-week period when changing from a SSRI to a MAOI. SSRIs, particularly Prozac, remain in the body for an extended period.

THE SELECTIVE SEROTONIN RE-UPTAKE INHIBITORS

Prozac (fluoxetine hydrochloride) was the first selective serotonin re-uptake inhibitor, or SSRI, put on the market. First introduced in 1987, it quickly became the most widely prescribed antidepressant medication ever. In fact, sales of Prozac accounted for $1.2 billion in 1995, and over 6 million Americans use it regularly. Prozac's success has spawned other SSRIs, including Zoloft (sertraline hydrochloride) and Paxil (paroxetine hydrochloride).

How do these drugs work? In Chapter 3, we saw how neurons release a neurotransmitter called serotonin into the synapses between cells. The SSRIs desensitize a receptor on the neuron that would normally absorb serotonin into the cell. As a result, there is a greater supply of serotonin in the synapse, which allows the neurons to transmit a stronger serotonin signal. Serotonin is one of the brain's natural antidepressants, so higher serotonin levels enhance mood and bring about a reduction in depressive symptoms.

The introduction of the SSRIs was considered a major advance in the pharmaceutical treatment of depression. Prior to this time, the only synthetic drugs on the market were the tricyclic drugs and the MAOIs. These options all have a variety of side effects, and persons using the MAO inhibitors also have to follow a restricted diet. That is why the development of the SSRIs was seen as a significant breakthrough.

Developed by Eli Lilly and Company after fifteen years of clinical research, Prozac has been marketed as a highly effective solution for depressive symptoms. It has even been recommended in bestselling books as a way to develop a more "socially rewarding personality." Yet despite all the media attention, studies show that Prozac is no more effective than St. John's wort—or other antidepressant drugs, for that matter—in combating depression.

Prozac and the other SSRIs can exact a high price for their benefits. Prozac is considered better than the older drugs because "only" 17 percent of the people who try it have to stop because of negative experiences, compared with nearly a third (31 percent) of the patients taking the tricyclic drugs. The reported side effects of Prozac, listed in percentage of incidence, include nausea (21 percent), headaches (20 percent), anxiety and nervousness (15 percent), insomnia (14 percent), drowsiness (12 percent), diarrhea (12 percent), dry mouth (9 percent), loss of appetite (9 percent), sweating and tremors (8 percent), and rashes (3 percent). In my own practice, and in reports from others, I believe these percentages are far too low, and that the true incidence of side effects is much higher. This discrepancy is likely due to the limited time span in the initial studies (only four to six weeks), and to the relatively small number of subjects.

The SSRIs also reduce sex drive. Studies that looked specifically at sexual dysfunction found that 34 percent of all men and women using Prozac had a drop in libido or difficulty in attaining orgasm. Again, in my experience, the figure is much higher. Many patients do not mention this as a side effect for a number of reasons, including embarrassment and the fact that sex simply isn't an issue for some people. For others, the loss of sex drive is balanced out by the reduction in depressive symptoms.

Prozac is also more likely than other antidepressants to cause restlessness and agitation. Some people have even experienced violent or destructive outbursts, and the drug's association with suicide remains controversial.

Zoloft and Paxil are similar to Prozac in terms of their side effects. However, Paxil tends to be more sedating, making it preferable for people with anxiety or insomnia. Zoloft generally falls in between the stimulating Prozac and the sedating Paxil, but individuals will differ in their responses.

The newest SSRI is Serzone (nefazodone hydrochloride), which is especially useful in cases of agitation, anxiety, and insomnia. Side effects were mild in a 2,200 patient sample, according to a manufacturer's premarketing trial. It appears to have the lowest incidence of sexual dysfunction of all the SSRIs, and also appears to be more effective in reducing suicide risk.

THE OTHER ANTIDEPRESSANTS

There are antidepressants that don't fall into any of the established classes: Wellbutrin, Desyrel, and Effexor.

Wellbutrin

Wellbutrin (bupropion hydrochloride) seems to boost norepinephrine function, with no impact on serotonin levels. Chemically related to amphetamine, it usually has a more energizing effect than the other synthetic drugs. Wellbutrin does not affect the heart or libido as do antidepressants, so it is often used to treat depression in individuals who have problems in these areas. It has also proved useful in the treatment of bipolar depression and a condition known as attention deficit disorder, which is characterized by impulsive behavior and a short attention span.

The main difficulty with this drug is its association with seizures. While this problem appears to be dosage related, Wellbutrin has been found to cause seizures in 1 in every 200 persons who take it. Psychiatrists tend to shy away from it for this reason, although a new timed-release version may eliminate this problem. Other side effects include restlessness, insomnia, irritability, and headache. Wellbutrin must be taken three times per day, another inconvenience, to maintain a relatively stable concentration level in the blood.

Desyrel

Desyrel (trazodone hydrochloride) works on the serotonin system. Rather than being used for its antidepressant effects, it is most often prescribed along with Prozac because the drowsiness Desyrel induces counteracts Prozac's tendency to produce insomnia. Desyrel's other side effects include headache, upset stomach, low blood pressure, dizziness, and dry mouth. In men, it can also cause a dangerous condition called priapism— painful, drug-induced erections that may not end upon discontinuing the drug. These side effects explain why Desyrel is seldom prescribed as an antidepressant.

Effexor

Effexor (venlafaxine hydrochloride) is chemically similar to an antidepressant compound in chocolate known as phenylethylamine (PEA), sometimes associated with the "love effect." It is likely that PEA raises the level of endorphins in the brain, which creates a sense of well-being. The tradition of giving chocolates on Valentine's Day reflects our intuitive knowledge of this effect.

Effexor is able to inhibit serotonin re-uptake as effectively as Prozac, yet it also boosts norepinephrine levels much as the tricyclic drugs do. That means it provides the benefits of the tricyclic medications without producing many of their side effects. Effexor also provides benefits for nearly half of the patients who do not respond to other antidepressant drugs, a far higher response rate than for other medications.

However, some 37 percent of the patients who try Effexor report problems with nausea, and one in every five persons experience dizziness, drowsiness, or dry mouth. Sleep disturbances can occur, as well. It can also increase blood pressure, so persons with high blood pressure should avoid the drug. On the good side, it does not seem to intensify the effects of tranquilizers or alcohol. It must be taken two or three times per day due to its short half-life, and dosages should be tapered off over two weeks to avoid withdrawal symptoms of severe rebound anxiety and depression. This can be extremely disabling, and sometimes even dangerous. I have seen suicidal depression result from sudden Effexor withdrawal.

THE PROBLEM OF SIDE EFFECTS

Scientific studies and the personal experiences of millions of patients have given us new insight into the frequent side effects produced by synthetic antidepressants. We now know that some of these medications can cause problems in up to a third of all users, forcing some to stop treatment altogether. We have also learned that particular classes of drugs are better tolerated than others. The MAOIs, for example, have fewer side effects than the tricyclics, but still produce multiple actions within the body that are unrelated to depression. These drugs can be particularly troublesome, even life-threatening, when taken in combination with certain foods or chemicals.

The reason for these side effects is related to the nature of synthetic drugs. When we affect one system in the body, we often affect others in both a positive and negative sense. For instance, a class of drugs called beta-blockers, commonly prescribed for high blood pressure, often adversely affect the brain's chemistry, causing depression. It simply isn't possible to isolate the brain biochemically from the circulatory system. Medications may have a single intended action, but it is impossible for them to not affect other parts of the body. This often creates unwanted, and sometimes dangerous, side effects (see *Talking Back to Prozac* in Appendix A). I have seen very severe toxic reactions to SSRIs—resulting in permanent damage—in susceptible individuals.

It may seem odd that drugs can produce a side effect in some individuals but not in others. Yet each of us has a unique brain and body biochemistry. For reasons that are still not totally understood, certain people respond better to one medication than another. They may have a more pronounced reduction in their depression, or not have any side effects to speak of. Another person could take the same dosage and have quite different results. Consequently, the selection of the best antidepressant medication is often a matter of an educated guess, followed by trial and error, for the psychiatrist.

For many people, particularly those who come to me for a change to St. John's wort, the side effects they experience are so intense—or the expense is so high—that they prefer to stop synthetic medications altogether. Jan, Jeremy, and Will can all attest to this.

> Jan: "I've suffered from dysthymia all my life. What worked for me was to drink a lot, until alcoholism stopped that dead in its tracks. Then came Prozac. It worked OK, but I couldn't stand the side effects. Then I took Zoloft for three months, 100 milligrams A.M. and 100 milligrams P.M. It worked. It cost a lot. I am also not sure I liked the leveling off of all my emotions! So, a month ago I began substituting St. John's wort, two tabs at night instead of the two doses of Zoloft. I'm very happy with the results. I no longer suffer debilitating PMS, either."

> Jeremy: "I was on Prozac for two years and just about went broke buying it. I then switched to Wellbutrin and that was much better on my pocketbook than Prozac. I then switched to St. John's wort, a German brand, at about $24 for sixty 300-milligram tablets. I then found out that I could get the same thing made in the States for seven dollars. That is where I am now, and I feel great! With no side effects at all!"

> Will: "My wife was on Prozac. It led her to have an 'I don't give a damn' attitude about important things, and to stomach distress the entire time she was on it. She then went off Prozac and started on St. John's wort. The stomach distress went away the day she stopped Prozac. Now that she's on her 'wart,' as she calls it, she is relaxed and cares about the important things in her life."

In many cases, besides the side effects, synthetic antidepressants produce subtle emotional results: complaints of flatness, of not caring, of dulled emotional responses. St. John's wort, in contrast, produces none of these effects. It not only counters the depressive feelings, but allows a natural brightness of emotion and sharpness of mental functioning to emerge.

That is why I prefer to use natural products such as herbs whenever possible. They have been used for thousands of years and have a much better safety record. In fact, when herbs do affect systems other than the targeted system, those extra effects are often positive in nature. Also, the multiple components in herbs are usually at a low enough concentration that they don't affect any one area too strongly. Their healing power is due to the synergistic effects produced by the combination of components. That is the very beauty of herbs. They promote balance and healing.

To summarize the benefits of St. John's wort when compared with synthetic antidepressants:

- Its side effects are not nearly as severe, and far less frequent.

- It does not have adverse effects when mixed with alcohol.

- It is nonaddictive.

- It does not produce withdrawal symptoms when you stop taking it.

- It does not produce habituation, or the need for increased dosages to maintain its effects.

- Its use can easily be restarted without requiring a long buildup period.

- It enhances sleep and dreaming.

- It does not produce daytime sedation. In fact, it has

shown experimentally to enhance alertness and driving reaction time.

• It does not produce agitation or instability.

According to one report, overdoses yielded an annual rate of 30.1 deaths per one million prescriptions of antidepressant. No one has ever died from an overdose of St. John's wort.

MAKING THE RIGHT DECISION

There is a role for both herbs and drugs in psychiatric treatment. There are circumstances when one or the other is called for, and there are situations when both are needed in combination. During my years of clinical practice, I have found that herbs should be the first line of defense. Their more gentle actions are often all that is needed to resolve the imbalances leading to depression. The more concentrated synthetic medications should be reserved for those times when their benefits outweigh their costs.

Synthetic antidepressants are highly purified, chemical substances that can provide many benefits, and can be a valuable resource in the treatment of severe depression and bipolar disorder. But they all have potentially harmful side effects. This is why a prescription is required from a psychiatrist or other medical practitioner. He or she is the one who can make an educated decision as to the best choice of drug. Your role as the patient is to be good observer and reporter, and to help guide this process, before and during treatment.

So far, as I've said, the value of St. John's wort has been proven only in the treatment of mild to moderate depression and seasonal affective disorder. While the herb may be an excellent adjunctive treatment for the treatment of major depression, there is not yet enough evidence to establish its usefulness as the sole medication for this disorder. I recommend that if you suffer from either major depression or bipolar disorder and want to use St. John's wort, you do so in consultation with a psychiatrist.

If you are dissatisfied with how your doctor responds to your questions about medications or herbs, I urge you to get a second opinion. I have heard many stories about patients who, after complaining of side effects to their doctors, were ignored or brushed off with "you can't possibly be having such side effects." Sometimes, doctors have even increased the dosage, which only aggravates the problem. Remember, your doctor isn't living inside *your* body. Only you know how you feel. You have a right to be heard, and to have your doctor work with you on fine-tuning your medication needs (see page 141).

I think you now understand why I always use St. John's wort as my first resort. This herb may not be able to help everyone, but it is unlikely to ever hurt anyone. Its side effects are always mild and temporary, and they occur far less frequently than with the other treatments. There are further considerations to keep in mind when you take St. John's wort. In the next chapter, I will discuss other natural supplements you can take to round out your treatment program.

8

Nutritional Approaches to Mental Health

Let food be thy medicine.

Hippocrates

Besides the oxygen we breathe, all that we need to survive comes from what we eat and drink. Food nourishes both the body and the brain. In fact, the brain has first call on the available supply of nutrients. Therefore, the first effects of nutritional deficiencies are often mental symptoms.

When orthomolecular psychiatrists refer to a nutritional deficiency, they are not necessarily talking about the prevention of a traditional deficiency disease, such as beriberi, a once-common illness that is fortunately now rare due to vitamin B_1 food supplementation. However, lesser *subclinical* deficiencies are quite common. While not enough to bring on overt physical symptoms, they are often sufficient to stimulate changes in brain chemistry, and affect mood. Antidepressants, including St. John's wort, are not likely to be successful in treating these cases until the specific deficiency is corrected.

In this chapter, I will introduce you to someone who was helped by nutritional therapy, and present information on vital depression-fighting nutrients. I'll then discuss other possible causes of depression—including illnesses that St. John's wort can help alleviate. (For information on the use of other herbs, see Chapter 5.)

TREATING THE ENTIRE PERSON

When treating depression, it is important to address all of a patient's problems, both biochemical and psychological, if healing is to take place. Jeff is a good example.

Jeff, a 19-year-old college freshman with no prior history of emotional problems, was brought to see me by his concerned father. "I don't know what to think. Jeff has been withdrawing more and more lately, won't join us at the dinner table, hasn't been finishing his assignments, and says there's nothing wrong." Further questioning revealed that Jeff had been popular in high school, a good student, and a member of the basketball team. Yet he was now failing at the local college he was attending, and according to his father, was "not his old self."

As his father talked, the tall, somewhat thin, young man sat across from me, looking sullen. I asked his father to leave the room so I could see Jeff alone. There was little change in his demeanor. A series of questions went through my mind: Was he depressed? Was he psychotic, hearing voices that he would not admit to? Or, putting on my orthomolecular hat, was he eating a typical teenage diet of fast food and soft drinks, which could leave him deficient in nutrients needed for adequate brain function?

I determined from his rather brief answers that he

was not in any immediate danger, but that he would need more time before he trusted me enough to talk more freely. Given his good prior history, I was willing to wait another week or so before doing anything more definitive, such as prescribing medication. My philosophy is "natural is preferable," since it addresses the root of the problem, and not the symptoms. Also, young people often feel stigmatized by a psychiatric diagnosis, especially when it is accompanied by a prescription.

Jeff agreed to take some daily vitamins, minerals, and herbs. When he came alone to see me two weeks later, he was far more communicative, and appeared to have gained some weight. He had indeed been going through a difficult time, with inner conflict about life issues that he had not had to deal with in high school. He was also feeling that he had let down his parents in some way by not being as competent, decisive, and independent as he expected himself to be. This confusion and depression is not unusual for first-year college students, who face a radical change from familiar high school surroundings. However, he admitted that he had been helped by my advice despite himself. While he had "resented my Dad's dragging me to some shrink," he had followed my instructions by taking the vitamins and herbs three times daily with meals. This instruction also assured that he would eat regularly, and likely, with the family. He said that the supplements seemed to calm his worried mind, and gave him energy and clarity at the same time. He turned out to be quite bright and articulate, in contrast to our initial contact.

What were these pills? The basic multivitamin/multimineral capsules are standard fare in my office, often restoring energy and emotional balance in depleted individuals. The herbs were St. John's wort, the herbal antidepressant, and kava-kava, a South Pacific herb used to help relieve stress (see Chapter 5). As his depression and anxiety lifted, Jeff was able to think more clearly, and began to seek my advice. Psychotherapy, or any learning, can take place much better when the brain is working properly. Any prior attempts at therapy with Jeff would probably have driven him further away. However, with the proper brain food, he was able to have some insight into his situation, and move in the direction of healing.

Jeff's moodiness might have been ignored by those around him, as friends and family of depressed people often rationalize that while something is not quite right, the person remains healthy in most respects. But sweeping these difficult issues under the carpet may lead to catastrophic consequences. Fortunately for Jeff, early intervention on several levels prevented his disturbance from becoming chronic.

NUTRITIONAL BALANCE AND DEPRESSION: AMINO ACIDS, VITAMINS, MINERALS, AND OTHER NUTRIENTS

Like Jeff's diet, the standard American diet is deficient in many of the nutrients we need to stay healthy, both physically and mentally. Specific diets are beyond the scope of this book, but we will cover some basic dietary guidelines in Chapter 9.

What causes these deficiencies? We need only consider the high-sugar, low-fiber, additive-preserved foods that many people consume on a regular basis, combined with the impaired absorption of nutrients that accompanies such poor nutrition. Many people simply do not get the important nutrients needed for good health. They are at once overfed and undernourished, and a poorly nourished body contains a malnourished brain.

In my own practice, I prefer to begin psychotherapy only after excluding an underlying physical cause. In fact, deficiencies in almost any of the vitamins and minerals can show up first as emotional or mental symptoms, such as depression, anxiety, or impaired memory and concentration. Because lab tests to determine specific deficiencies can be costly, I most often recommend the use of multivitamin/multimineral supplements. (For more information on vitamins and minerals, see *Prescription for Nutritional Healing* and *The Real Vitamin and Mineral Book* in Appendix A.)

Let's look at the amino acids, vitamins, minerals, and other nutrients that are especially important for mental health. (The essential fatty acids are also significant in the prevention and treatment of depression and other disorders; they are discussed in Chapter 9.)

Amino Acids

As we saw in Chapter 3, depression can result if brain messengers called neurotransmitters are in short supply. Synthetic antidepressants work by raising neurotransmitter levels in the brain, and it is likely that St. John's wort does the same thing. Amino acids, the building blocks of protein, are the *precursors*, or raw materials, for neurotransmitters and other mood-regulating compounds. It is possible to reverse depression by loading up on these amino-acid precursors.

There are three amino acids that are most directly related to mood and depression: phenylalanine, tyrosine, and tryptophan. Phenylalanine and tyrosine produce the neurotransmitter norepinephrine, and tryptophan is eventually converted to serotonin.

Research has proven the effectiveness of amino acid therapy in fighting depression. Both phenylalanine and tyrosine—which is created in the body from phenylalanine—have been found to be as effective as the antidepressant drug imipramine. Phenylalanine has also been shown to reduce pain by preserving brain levels of endorphins, the body's natural painkiller. Tyrosine is helpful in the treatment of PMS and chronic fatigue syndrome (see page 127). Tryptophan, which the body converts into the precursor 5-hydroxytryptophan (5-HT), has also been found to be as effective as the synthetic antidepressants.

Since amino acids are found in such high-protein foods as meat, fish, and eggs, you might think that the way to increase your amino-acid levels would be to eat more of these foods. However, disorders such as depression are caused by specific amino-acid imbalances. I recommend that you work with your physician to determine which amino acids you are deficient in before undertaking a supplementation program (see *The Way Up From Down* in Appendix A). If you are already taking antidepressant medication, you can keep taking it while your biochemistry is being brought into balance, and then discontinue the medication after the amino acid therapy takes effect. Amino acids can be combined with St. John's wort. It is important to take sufficient amounts of the amino-acid cofactors, such as vitamin B_6, which your body needs to properly process amino acids. Tryptophan is available only by prescription at compounding pharmacies, or pharmacies that carry natural medicines, but 5-HT is now available from a limited number of suppliers. I still recommend that amino acid therapy be carried out under professional supervision, to insure correct product and dosage.

Vitamins

Our bodies cannot create vitamins, so a well-balanced, supplemented diet is necessary to obtain adequate amounts of these essential nutrients. Vitamins act as catalytic agents in the body, helping to speed up the chemical processes that are vital for both survival and brain function. As a result, vitamin deficiencies can sometimes manifest themselves as depression. Fortunately, when these deficiencies are treated with supplements, there is a reversal in symptoms.

The Recommended Daily Allowance (RDA) is inadequate. These figures are based on the minimal requirements for prevention of severe deficiency disease, rather than on the requirements for optimum health or deficiency correction. My recommendations exceed the RDA. For vitamins B_1, B_3, and B_6, I recommend a daily dose of 50 milligrams (mg), with higher doses for specific disorders.

Important vitamins for mental health include:

- *Vitamin B_1 (thiamine)*. The brain uses this vitamin to help convert glucose, or blood sugar, into fuel, and without it the brain rapidly runs out of energy. This can lead to fatigue, depression, irritability, anxiety, and even thoughts of suicide. Deficiencies can also cause memory problems, loss of appetite, insomnia, and gastrointestinal disorders. The consumption of refined carbohydrates, such as simple sugars, drains the body's B_1 supply.

- *Vitamin B_3 (niacin)*. As we saw in Chapter 3, pellagra—which produces psychosis and dementia, among other symptoms—was eventually found to be caused by niacin deficiency. Many commercial food products now contain niacin, and pellagra has virtually disappeared. However, subclinical deficiencies of vitamin B_3 can produce agitation and anxiety, as well as mental and physical slowness. Megadoses of the vitamin have been found to reduce these symptoms.

- *Vitamin B₆ (pyridoxine)*. This nutrient is essential for the creation of neurotransmitters. Studies have found a strong correlation between vitamin B_6 deficiency and depression. Shortages can also produce anemia, numbness, tingling in the limbs, and convulsions. Vitamin B_6 has been shown to help women with premenstrual syndrome (PMS). Malabsorption diseases and certain drugs, including MAOI antidepressants (see Chapter 7) and birth control pills, can cause deficiencies. I recommend that all women on birth control pills take 50 mg of vitamin B_6 daily.

- *Vitamin B₁₂ (cobalamin)*. Because vitamin B_{12} is important to red blood cell formation, deficiency leads to an oxygen-transport problem known as pernicious anemia. This disorder can cause mood swings, paranoia, irritability, confusion, dementia, hallucinations, or mania, eventually followed by appetite loss, dizziness, weakness, shortage of breath, heart palpitations, diarrhea, and tingling sensations in the extremities. Deficiencies take a long time to develop, since the body stores a three- to five-year supply in the liver. When shortages do occur, they are often due to a lack of intrinsic factor, an enzyme that allows vitamin B_{12} to be absorbed in the intestinal tract. Since intrinsic factor diminishes with age, older people are more prone to B_{12} deficiencies. Thus, this vitamin is often given as an injection, or as tablets that dissolve under the tongue, to bypass the digestive tract. Vitamin B_{12} can benefit the 10 to 30 percent of depressed individuals who are deficient. The dose is 1,000 micrograms (mcg).

- *Folic acid (folate)*. Folic acid, another B vitamin, helps assist in the creation of many neurotransmitters. It is also essential to the production of hemoglobin, the oxygen-bearing substance in red blood cells, so deficiencies often lead to anemia. Studies have shown abnormally low levels of this vitamin in from a quarter to a third of all depressed persons. Other symptoms include fatigue, lower-extremity problems, and dementia. Orthomolecular psychiatrists have used folic acid supplements for many years to reduce the frequency of relapses in their patients. Poor dietary habits contribute to folic acid deficiencies, as do illness, alcoholism, and various drugs, including aspirin, birth control pills, barbiturates, and anticonvulsants. It is usually administered along with vitamin B_{12}, since the folic acid can mask a deficiency of B_{12}. The usual dose is 800 mcg. Higher doses, though safe, require a prescription.

- *Vitamin C (ascorbic acid).* Vitamin C, widely known for its antioxidant abilities, is also important for mental health. Subclinical deficiencies can produce depression, which requires the use of supplements. One study showed that a single 3-gram dose of vitamin C reduced symptoms by 40 percent in eleven manic and twelve depressed patients after only four hours. Supplementation is particularly important if you have had surgery or an inflammatory disease. Stress, pregnancy, and lactation also increase the body's need for vitamin C, while aspirin, tetracycline, and birth control pills can deplete the body's supply. A good maintenance dose is 1 to 3 grams daily, with more for depressed people, smokers, and those exposed to toxins of various kinds.

Minerals

There are at least fifteen minerals that are essential to health. Either inadequate or excessive dietary intake can lead to mental and behavioral problems, including depression, often before any physical symptoms appear.

Minerals important to mental health include:

- *Sodium and potassium.* These minerals are considered together because they determine the body's electrolyte balance, which regulates water levels. Eating a lot of salty food (sodium) disrupts this balance. This not only produces high blood pressure, but also affects neurotransmitter levels, producing depression and PMS. In addition, the misuse of diuretics, or "water pills," can lead to potassium deficiency, which in turn can manifest itself as depression. A good daily dose is from 200 to 400 mg.

- *Iron.* Iron deficiency can result in anemia, which can produce symptoms such as depression, irritability, fatigue, loss of attention span, and insomnia. One study found that nearly half of all premenopausal women and a third of all children do not get enough iron, so supplementation in these groups could have a significant impact on the frequency of depression and other disorders. From 15 to 30 mg a day is a good maintenance dose. On the other hand, excessive iron can lead to toxicity, especially in men, who are not losing the mineral regularly through menstruation. Therefore, men shouldn't supplement with iron unless under a doctor's direction.

- *Magnesium.* This mineral assists in all of the body's energy reactions. Deficiency can result in depressive symptoms, along with confusion, agitation, anxiety, and hallucinations, as well as a variety of physical problems. Most diets do not include enough magnesium, and stress also contributes to magnesium depletion. Other possible reasons for a deficiency include kidney or parathyroid disease, high blood pressure, chronic fluid loss, alcoholism, and malabsorption disorders. Several studies have shown that magnesium injections can bring relief from symptoms such as fatigue, aches and pains, weakness, and lethargy. I frequently give magnesium shots for migraine headaches, PMS, and allergies. A daily maintenance dose is 400 to 800 mg, with more needed to correct deficiencies.

• *Calcium.* Depressed individuals often have excessive calcium levels, particularly those with bipolar disorder (see Chapter 2). When these patients recover, their calcium levels usually return to normal. Depression can also occur in cases of calcium deficiency, long before the appearance of physical deficiency symptoms. In addition, calcium works with magnesium to maintain balance, or homeostasis, in the body, much as sodium and potassium work together to achieve balance in water levels. If you are supplementing with calcium, you will need to take one-half as much magnesium, sometimes even more, to keep the two properly balanced. This includes women who are taking calcium supplements to prevent osteoporosis. A good daily dose is 800 to 1,000 mg.

• *Zinc.* Zinc deficiencies frequently lead to depression, since this mineral is essential to many processes related to brain function. In addition to irritability, mental slowness, and emotional disorders, zinc deficiency can produce changes in taste and smell sensations, a loss of appetite, reduced immune function, and rough skin. These symptoms are particularly common among older people and in women, especially those with eating disorders. An excellent treatment for anorexia and bulimia uses high doses of zinc, beyond the recommended 15 to 30 mg daily.

Other Nutrients

There are two other nutrients that are important to mental health. *S-adenosylmethionine* (SAM), a natural, active form of the amino acid methionine, helps process a wide variety of neurotransmitters, including norepinephrine, dopamine, phosphatidylcholine, serotonin, and melatonin. In Europe, SAM is sold as an antidepressant, where it performs as well or better than synthetic drugs without the side effects.

Phosphatidylserine, another substance that is particularly plentiful in the brain, helps to ensure proper nerve function by keeping the membrane surrounding each brain cell fluid and flexible. Proper membrane fluidity affects nerve signal transmission, the binding of neurotransmitters to receptor sites, and the activity of monoamine oxidase, or MAO (see Chapter 3). Phosphatidylserine can also enhance mood, behavior, and mental function by increasing the accumulation, storage, and release of several neurotransmitters. I have used it successfully in my practice as an adjunct in treating depression and to improve cognitive functions such as thinking and memory, in doses of 100 mg two to three times a day. It should *not* be combined with an antidepressant without a doctor's supervision, nor is it recommended for bipolar disorder (see Chapter 2).

OTHER POSSIBLE CAUSES OF DEPRESSION

There are several illnesses that can mimic depression, including chronic fatigue syndrome, systemic candidiasis, and hypoglycemia, or low blood sugar. St. John's wort can be especially useful in treating the first two disorders; both are related to immune dysfunction, and St. John's wort can fight depression and strengthen the immune system (see Chapter 4). Two additional factors to consider in depression are hormonal imbalances and the effects of pollution. (See *Solving the Puzzle of Chronic Fatigue Syndrome* in Appendix A.)

Chronic Fatigue Syndrome

Chronic fatigue syndrome (CFS) is an often-baffling disorder that can thoroughly disrupt someone's life, as Melissa discovered.

Melissa, a successful 38-year-old professional, described herself in desperate terms: "I feel like I'm losing my mind. I'm absent-minded, simple tasks overwhelm me, and I'm in tears at the drop of a hat. I'm exhausted most of the time. I can barely get up in the morning. All day, there's a constant struggle to stay awake. I feel my life is over!"

Melissa's medical history revealed unaddressed explanations for her desperation. Six months earlier, she'd had the flu. Despite her apparent recovery after about a month, she never fully regained her former strength and energy. She could no longer exercise as before, and found that it depleted rather than energized her. She drank coffee to boost her energy, but after a while even that did not work.

I ordered several blood tests. They revealed a number of problems, any one of which could cause fatigue, anxiety, and depression: iron-deficiency anemia, elevated Epstein-Barr viral antibodies—which indicated both a past and presently active viral infection—and hypoglycemia. I prescribed an iron supplement for the anemia, a standard medical diagnosis that is often overlooked. However, in contrast to standard treatment, I also prescribed immune-boosting and energizing herbs, including astragalus, echinacea, goldenseal, licorice, and Siberian ginseng. In addition, Melissa took St. John's wort, megadoses of vitamins and minerals, and specific amino acids, especially lysine and cysteine, for viral defense. Within three months she was feeling like herself again—active, enthusiastic, optimistic, and no longer depressed.

Melissa's flu turned out to be Epstein-Barr virus, a chronic, relapsing form of infectious mononucleosis that is part of CFS. CFS appears to be caused by any one of a group of viruses that can lie dormant for months or years at a time, then be reactivated by physical or emotional stress. Symptoms include depression, extreme fatigue, nonrestorative sleep, impaired memory and concentration, anxiety attacks, intermittent low-grade fevers, sore throat, swollen lymph glands, muscle aches and pains, and allergies. One feature that distinguishes CFS from depression or other causes of fatigue is a negative response to exercise. While most individuals feel energized after exercise, chronic fatigue patients feel worse.

Systemic Candidiasis (Candida Infection)

Systemic candidiasis is caused by the fungus *Candida albicans*, an organism normally found in the intestines and elsewhere that can grow out of control under certain conditions. Joni is a good example of how candidiasis can affect mood.

> *Joni, an overweight, depressed, 32-year-old secretary, was in tears. "Everything I eat makes my stomach bloat like I'm six months' pregnant. I keep dieting, and I can't lose weight. My brain is like mush: I'm absent-minded, and afraid I'm going to lose my job. Yesterday, I went to get coffee for my boss, went to the file drawer instead, and couldn't remember what I was doing!" She craved sugar and bread, and had repeated vaginal yeast infections and severe PMS. She scored high on a candida questionnaire, and a candida antibody blood test confirmed the diagnosis.*
>
> *Joni had taken antibiotics as a teenager to combat acne. This set her up for overgrowth of yeast in the intestinal tract. She had also started taking birth control*

pills at the age of twenty-four, leading to a hormonal state that favors candida growth. Fortunately, she responded well to treatment, which included a healthy diet, two acidophilus capsules a half hour before each meal, and two tannic acid capsules taken three times daily. Her abdominal bloating cleared, as did her PMS, mood swings, and mental fogginess. She was finally able to lose weight, as well.

Systemic candidiasis, also known as chronic *Candida albicans* or candida hypersensitivity syndrome, is similar to CFS in its effects. *Candida albicans* is normally kept in balance within the gastrointestinal tract by the friendly bacteria that aid in digestion, such as acidophilus. If these friendly bacteria are weakened, candida can start to overgrow, causing a multitude of symptoms that are often erroneously labelled psychosomatic.

As in Joni's case, long-term use of antibiotics kills the body's friendly bacteria, making it easier for candida to overgrow. When used with steroids, antibiotics also suppress the immune system. Repeated pregnancies and prolonged use of either birth control pills or progesterone can change the body's hormonal balance, which can also lead to candidiasis. A diet high in sugar will promote candida growth, both because the yeast grows on sugar and because sugar has an immune-suppressant effect.

Like CFS, candidiasis is a controversial diagnosis in orthodox medical circles, usually acknowledged only in severely debilitated patients. For more information on this subject, see *The Yeast Connection* and *The Yeast Syndrome* in Appendix A.

Hypoglycemia

Melissa, the patient with CFS, also had hypoglycemia.

This disorder is often related both to stress and to poor eating habits, both of which affect the adrenal glands. As we saw in Chapter 3, our adrenal glands produce hormones that allow us to deal with emergencies. One of these hormones, cortisol, raises blood-sugar levels temporarily. After a while, though, blood-sugar levels plummet. When this cycle repeats itself enough, the overtaxed adrenal glands are exhausted—and so are we.

Hypoglycemia can present itself in a variety of ways: depression, irritability, anxiety, panic attacks, fatigue, "brain fog," headaches (including migraines), insomnia, muscular weakness, and tremors, all of which may be relieved by food. There can be cravings for sweets, coffee, alcohol, or drugs; in fact, many addictions are related to hypoglycemia. In Melissa's case, in addition to the CFS therapy, I prescribed a diet in which sugar, white flour, coffee, and alcohol were to be eliminated, and replaced by small, frequent meals containing complex carbohydrates, high fiber, and protein. (For more information on hypoglycemia, see Chapter 9.)

Hormonal Imbalances and Pollution Effects

Imbalances in either sex or thyroid hormones can cause depression. Sex hormone imbalances are more common in women because of the complications presented by the menstrual cycle, as we can see in Lonnie's case.

Lonnie, a 40-year-old secretary, was still depressed, anxious, irritable, and tired despite six months of weekly therapy sessions, after which her therapist had referred her to me. Lonnie was dissatisfied with her job, her family, and life in general, and had severe PMS. Blood tests showed that she was perimenopausal, that time period prior to menopause when hormone levels are already beginning to change.

I prescribed the female herbal remedies dong quai, vitex, and black cohosh. I also had her take two hormones, natural progesterone and dehydroepiandrosterone (DHEA), plus vitamin B_6, magnesium, and evening primrose oil. Considering her level of depression and anxiety, I added St. John's wort and kava, both noted for their effects on PMS and menopausal symptoms. After about six weeks on this regimen, not only did her PMS go away, but so did her depression and irritability. Her energy level and sexual response both improved. We see how in Lonnie's case, addressing the physical problem had a positive effect on her emotions.

Natural hormone therapy is far more preferable than the usual synthetic hormone replacement therapy. Unlike the synthetic hormones, natural progesterone and estrogen have few side effects, and are available at compounding pharmacies. See Appendix A for books on the subject, and Appendix B for names of compounding pharmacies.

Low levels of thyroid hormone, produced by the energy-generating gland located below the Adam's apple, can also cause depression, as in Randi's case.

When Randi, a 34-year-old guidance counselor, came to see me, she was depressed, tired, unable to get up in the morning, and feeling overwhelmed by her job. She was often cold, especially her hands and feet. She also had thinning hair, dry skin, and constipation. When I asked about thyroid disease, she said that it had been suspected before, but her tests had been normal. An underactive thyroid, however, can often hide behind "normal" blood tests. Although Randi's thyroid hormone levels were normal, she did, in fact, have hypothyroidism, or low thyroid function. I pre-

scribed thyroid hormone from natural sources and asked her to monitor her body temperature so I could adjust her dosage. She asked whether this would suppress her own thyroid function and whether she would need supplementation for life. The answer was "no" to both questions. The treatment actually supported her own thyroid gland, allowing it to heal. Within ten days of starting the program, Randi's mood and energy lifted, and she was feeling alive again.

Dr. Broda Barnes has developed a technique of monitoring thyroid function through body temperature that is used by many alternative health practitioners. If the temperature is consistently low, the patient is treated with thyroid replacement therapy, and progress is monitored both by clinical signs and symptoms, and by a rise in temperature (see *Hypothyroidism* in Appendix A).

Depression can be caused by a wide variety of pollutants, especially the heavy metals: lead, mercury, arsenic, and bismuth. Aluminum, though technically not a heavy metal, is also toxic. Other pollutants can cause problems, too. Carbon monoxide reduces the brain's oxygen supply, which causes a variety of psychiatric and neurological symptoms, including psychotic depression. Insecticide exposure can result in depression, confusion, drowsiness, and decreased concentration. Other volatile substances, such as paint and solvents, can also result in depression and other psychiatric symptoms when the fumes are inhaled for prolonged periods of time. The best way to avoid exposure to pollutants is to minimize your risks (see *Our Stolen Future* in Appendix A).

The psychiatrist can be not only a healer, but an educator and facilitator as well, helping people to make wise choices in lifestyle, diet, supplements, and medications. Rather than curing depression, the goal is balance, in body as well as in mind and spirit. Imbalance in one area is reflected in problems in other areas, and the weakest link shows first. Ideal treatment is wholistic: Evaluate the whole person and treat each imbalance accordingly. Address as many areas—physical, emotional, and spiritual—as possible, thereby encouraging shifts that move the individual toward balance and health. With that in mind, I will provide some guidelines for living a depression-free lifestyle in the next chapter.

9

Living a Depression-Free Lifestyle

As we've seen, depression does not "just happen." While genetics and early history are contributing factors, depression often reflects poor lifestyle choices, including inadequate diet, lack of exercise, high stress, smoking, alcohol and drug abuse, and excessive caffeine consumption. You cannot take a pill and overcome a lifetime of poor health habits.

The foundation of a depression-free lifestyle consists of a good diet, a regular exercise and stress-reduction program, and elimination of addictions. Don't worry about willpower; this chapter does not contain power-through-the-pain types of advice. You will find that you do not have to be a fanatic about your behavior, that baby steps count, and that healthy living is its own reward.

A HEALTHY DIET FOR A HEALTHY MIND

A healthy diet consists of two parts: eating the right foods, and dealing with foods that provoke allergies.

Eating for Health

How, then, shall you eat? On a 1,500-calorie-a-day limit? For your blood type? Grapefruit before 10 A.M. and pasta at noon? The diet world presents a difficult maze to navigate. I will cover some of the basic information, including several of the more popular trends, and give overall guidelines for healthy eating.

In Chapter 8, we discussed the micronutrients: amino acids, vitamins, and minerals. These are fine-tuning elements, the cofactors that help convert our food into tissue and energy. The bulk of our diet consists of the macronutrients: carbohydrates, proteins, and fats.

Carbohydrates, such as cereals, grains, breads, and vegetables, can be rated by their *glycemic index*. This index measures how quickly a specific food is turned into glucose, or blood sugar, which in turn stimulates the pancreas to release insulin. High glycemic foods, such as doughnuts and candy, raise blood-glucose levels rapidly, which results in a large, fast release of insulin. Insulin removes sugar from the system and stores it as fat and glycogen. This causes your blood-glucose levels to drop, which makes you feel weak and lightheaded, and even cranky. Actually, you are hypoglycemic, or prone to low blood-sugar levels. The solution is to eat low glycemic foods, such as fruits and vegetables. These foods are turned into glucose more slowly, allowing for more stable blood-glucose levels and for greater energy levels. People who follow a Zone type of diet (see page 138), which helps to normalize blood-sugar levels, report increased stamina and stress-bearing ability, plus more stable moods. Carbohydrates also raise serotonin levels, which in this case leads to relaxation (see *The Serotonin Solution* in Appendix A).

Proteins, such as meat, fish, and eggs, are the building blocks of all bodily components, from hair and muscles to enzymes and hormones. They supply the precursors of neurotransmitters that increase alertness. So it's a good idea to start the day with a protein-based breakfast. Excessive protein intake, however, does encourage fat storage. In addition, it can also lead to *ketosis*, in which muscle tissue is broken down to produce glucose for the brain; to osteoporosis; kidney disease; and heart disease.

Fats, such as oil and butter, are not always the dietary bad guys. The popularity of very low- to no-fat diets in recent years have actually contributed to a whole host of problems, from premenstrual syndrome (PMS) and infertility to depression and anxiety. A major problem is that most people don't recognize that certain fats are vital to health. These *essential fatty acids* produce hormones called eicosonoids, which are necessary for many chemical processes within the body. They stimulate the immune system, fight inflammation, and support the activity of neurotransmitters, including serotonin (see *Omega-3 Oils* in Appendix A).

Most of the currently popular diets, including the Zone, recommend minimizing your intake of saturated fat, such as that found in butter, eggs, and fatty meat, as well as your intake of the trans-fatty acids, such as those found in margarine. Instead, they recommend olive oil, canola oil, and polyunsaturated vegetable oils. While these recommendations are valid, egg whites do in fact contain high-quality protein, and the much-maligned yolks contain cholesterol, which in fact is essential for production of all the steroid hormones, among other things. Fertile eggs from range-fed, organically raised chickens, eaten lightly boiled or poached, provide an excellent source of protein and "good" fat. Another source of quality protein and fat are *raw*, unpasteurized dairy products from a certified dairy that uses no antibiotics or hormones. These healthful products contain enzymes that allow them to be readily broken down and assimilated within the body, and thus less likely to cause allergic reactions (see page 140).

In the past ten years, Americans have reduced their fat intake and increased their carbohydrate intake—and gained weight. There has also been a rise in the rates of arthritis, heart disease, and cancer. What is going on? Dr. Barry Sears, author of *Mastering the Zone* (see Appendix A), believes that this dietary shift to carbohydrates has contributed to the rise in health problems. He recommends that people reduce their carbohydrate intake while increasing their fat and protein intake, in a 40 percent to 30 percent to 30 percent ratio of carbohydrates, proteins, and fats, respectively.

Widely recognized nutritionist and author Anne Louise Gittleman has refined this concept by replacing some of the foods Sears recommends with more nutritious and natural foods, and by focusing on micronutrient content (see her *40-30-30 Diet* in Appendix A). She also explains the blood-type diet theory found in Peter D'Adamo's *Eat Right for Your Type* (see Appendix A). According to this theory, your ancestry, as marked by your blood type, determines which foods are best for you. This information allows you to discover personalized solutions for chronic weight problems, food allergies, and other diet-related conditions.

In essence, to follow a healthy diet, you should:

- Eat lots of fresh, organic fruits and vegetables. They provide vitamins, minerals, antioxidants, and other substances that protect against degenerative disease. They are rich in fragile components that diminish with time and exposure to air. Processed vegetables, on the other hand, may list all the correct nutrients on the label, but lack the vitality-giving properties of freshly picked produce. Avoid chemically grown produce. We are already overloaded with toxins, so why ingest more?

- Avoid processed foods. Not only are they devoid of "life force," but they contain dangerous additives. For example, the artificial sweetener aspartame is known to be toxic to the brain. I have seen many people whose severe anxiety and even bizarre behavior cleared up when they stopped drinking aspartame-containing diet soft drinks.

- Eliminate white flour and sugar, and other high glycemic, empty-calorie foods that cause weight gain and hypoglycemia and can promote the development of systemic candidiasis (see Chapter 8).

- Eat seeds, nuts, and whole grains, which haven't had all their nutrients stripped away.

- Reduce your overall fat intake. Avoid saturated fats and fried food. Instead, eat foods rich in essential fatty acids, such as flax, soy, pumpkin, and walnut oils, and cold-water fish such as salmon and mackerel.

- Avoid sources of caffeine, such as coffee, tea, and cola drinks.

- Limit alcohol consumption to one drink (4 ounces of wine) per day.

- Drink at least eight glasses of pure water a day. Considering that our bodies are 65 percent water, we must not ignore this life-giving element. According to Dr. F. Batmanghelidj, many health problems—including depression, high blood pressure, ulcers, and diabetes—respond to adequate amounts of water (see *Your Body Cries for Water* in Appendix A). Tap water is full of chlorine and fluoride, neither of which is good for you. Use filtered water. The two best processes are reverse osmosis and steam distillation, but they are also the bulkiest and most expensive. Other choices are bottled water, a carbon filter, or a ceramic filter.

Food and Chemical Sensitivities

We generally associate allergies with rashes, hives, nasal congestion, or gastrointestinal problems. However, food and chemical sensitivities can produce a great variety of symptoms, such as depression, anxiety, "brain fog," fatigue, hyperactivity, attention deficit disorder, joint pains, migraine headaches, and food cravings, mimicking many other diseases in the process. As a result, these sensitivities are often misdiagnosed, and may even be mislabelled as psychosomatic or hypochondriacal.

Alternative health practitioners, on the other hand, recognize food and chemical sensitivities for what they are, and recommend specific diagnostic and treatment programs. A common approach is "rotation and elimination," whereby the patient avoids the offending substance, then gradually reintroduces it until it is tolerated. This food can then be eaten on a rotating basis, no more than every four days, to avoid further sensitivity. The disadvantages of this technique include nutritional limitations, personal inconvenience, and the difficulty of avoiding common substances. After seeing so many people despair of finding a workable solution to this problem, I looked around for an easier alternative—and found it.

There is a simple desensitization technique called Nambudripad's Allergy Elimination Technique (NAET), named for the southern California doctor who developed it. It employs a diagnostic technique called applied kinesiology, in which an indicator muscle is used to determine if a particular substance causes weakness in the person's energy field. Acupuncture or acupressure is used to treat the weakness. After twenty-five hours, the patient can often resume eating the offending food or be exposed to the chemical without further problems. While this sounds unlikely, the results are compelling, and it helps to remember that Westerners were very skeptical of acupuncture itself when they first heard of it. If you are interested in NAET, consult an alternative health practitioner, or see *Say Good-bye to Illness* in Appendix A. (If you want to find an alternative health care practitioner, see Appendix B and read "How to Find an Understanding Doctor.")

How to Find an Understanding Doctor

Not all psychiatrists and physicians understand the roles that nutrient deficiencies and toxicities can play in depression. These are generally the same professionals who do not take a wholistic approach to medicine in general. Many still believe that depression is all in your mind, although an ever-growing number of doctors in all specialties are coming to realize the importance of nutrition in proper brain functioning.

If your family physician is open to wholistic medicine, he or she would be an obvious first choice, given his or her knowledge of your past medical history, as well as an on-going relationship with you. Your doctor may be familiar with the benefits of St. John's wort and other aspects of natural medicine, and may be willing to explore these possibilities. He or she may also know practitioners—psychiatrists, naturopaths, or others—who can conduct the detailed testing needed to find the nutritional deficiencies or toxicities that may be contributing to your depression. Be aware that few conventionally trained doctors are experts in the field of nutrition, and unfortunately, some who are not have jumped on this newly popular bandwagon. Membership in organizations of alternative physicians should start your screening process.

A psychiatrist is a medical doctor who has taken additional training in the form of a three- or four-year residency program. He or she learns diagnosis and treatment of mental and emotional illness, psychotherapy, biological aspects of mind and emotions, and psychopharmacology, or the use of medication for psychiatric conditions. Psychiatrists tend to treat more serious problems, and prescribe medication. Most therapy is carried out by psychotherapists and psychologists, who are familiar with the signs and symptoms of depression, and know when to refer a patient to a psychiatrist. While some therapists may be familiar with a nutritional approach, their licenses do not allow them to prescribe even nutritional supplements. On the other hand, orthomolecular psychiatrists, who look for underlying chemical imbalances and medical conditions in the treatment of mental illness, can and do prescribe nutritional supplements.

A psychiatrist may not be necessary in the alternative treatment of depression. If there is an imbalance present, any orthomolecular physician, either a doctor of medicine (M.D.) or doctor of osteopathy (D.O.), can diagnose and treat it. Osteopathic physicians receive training similar to that of conventional doctors, with the addition of spinal manipulation techniques and nutrition. However, in their desire to be accepted as scientific, many neglect their natural medicine training and favor synthetic drugs.

Other practitioners deal with various aspects of wholistic medicine. Naturopaths (N.D.s) study natural medicine in four-year accredited programs. Unfortunately, they are not yet licensed in all states. As a group, they are making an enormous contribution to research and education in the field of natural medicine, with such eminent teachers and authors as Joseph Pizzorno and Michael Murray. Doctors of Oriental medicine (O.M.D.s) are licensed in all states to practice herbal medicine and acupuncture. By itself, acupuncture can be an excellent way of regulating the imbalances that often underlie depression. Chiropractors (doctors of chiropractic, or D.C.s) can also be of help, if properly trained in clinical nutrition and the subtler forms of healing. Many, however, have limited their practices to spinal manipulation.

Nutritionists are varied in their training and experience, and should each be taken on their own skills, the recommendations of others, and their affiliation with medical practitioners and psychiatrists, to whom they refer patients when appropriate. I certainly have had excellent relationships with nutritionists in which we refer freely back and forth. Herbalists, like nutritionists, vary in their training and skills. Their background is more grassroots, coming from traditional folk medicine. The American Herbalists Guild is a well-respected organization whose membership is by invitation and peer review.

It is of greatest importance that you like and trust your health care professional. You should feel both free to ask questions and confident that you are being taken seriously. The relationship is a sacred one, based on the ancient tradition of priest-healer. A good part of the healing process is based in this very relationship. Trust your own intuition, both in terms of with whom you choose to work, and in which direction that person takes you.

A good doctor will pay attention to your ideas and be willing to learn from you, as well. This is a new model, a partnership in healing. Your doctor is the resource, the expert, in medical information and practice, and you are the expert in how you feel. The idea is to respect each other's roles in this relationship, and to each do your part.

STRESS REDUCTION AND EXERCISE
FOR A CALM MIND

Now that you know what to eat, let's look at areas of exercise and stress reduction.

Exercise: Stress Relief and Much More

Most people are aware of the physical benefits of exercise: heart-lung conditioning, weight control, bone and joint strengthening. But exercise also improves mood by producing positive biochemical changes in the body and brain. Regular exercise reduces the amount of adrenal hormones your body releases in response to stress (see Chapter 3). Also, exercise causes your body to release greater amounts of powerful, mood-elevating endorphins, producing the sensation known as "runner's high."

There have been over a hundred clinical studies examining the link between endorphins and exercise. One of the most interesting was conducted by Dr. Dennis Lobstein at the University of New Mexico. He compared ten men who jogged with ten sedentary men in the same age range. He discovered that the sedentary men were more depressed and had lower levels of endorphins, along with higher levels of stress hormones and higher perceived levels of stress in their lives. Other studies have since established that exercise, as an antidepressant, can be as effective as drugs and traditional psychotherapy. You do not have to be a seasoned athlete to benefit from endorphins, although the more intensely you exercise, the more you produce.

If you have never exercised before, and especially if you have a preexisting health condition, see your doctor before you begin. Then, start your exercise program gradually, such as with a walk around the block. Build up over time to a slow jog, first around the block, or a track, slowly increasing the distance and speed. Build up to a full jog that lasts between twenty and thirty minutes, several times a week.

Jogging, bicycling, swimming, and calisthenics are all forms of *aerobic exercise*, which conditions the heart and lungs. Weight lifting is an example of *resistance exercise*, which builds the muscles. It also counters osteoporosis, since bone development is stimulated by weight-bearing exercise. Both types of exercise are important to overall health. Also, all exercise takes your mind off your worries; think of the times when you played basketball, volleyball, jump rope, or tag with your friends.

No matter what activities you choose, keep the following tips in mind:

- Wear loose, comfortable clothing and comfortable sneakers.

- Warm up before exercise, use a lot of stretches, and cool down afterwards.

- Do not fall into the "pain is good" trap. Some muscular soreness or tightness is normal, but pain is a sign that something's wrong. If you hurt, and the pain persists, stop exercising and see your health practitioner.

- Don't overdo it, especially at the beginning. Rest between exercise sessions.

- Do something you enjoy. The more you enjoy an exercise, the more likely you are to stick with it.

Exercise can increase self-esteem. It is tangible evidence of your desire to improve yourself, and to take charge of your life. You can extend this realization to other aspects of your existence.

How to Keep Stress From Controlling Your Life

Stress, with its accompanying anxiety and tension, seems inevitable, but it takes a serious toll on our mental and physical health. Among its negative effects, chronic stress produces hormones such as cortisol that reduce immune-system function, as we saw in Chapter 3. A personal stress-reduction program is essential, especially if you are prone to depression.

We all experience stress. The other day, for example, I found myself on line at the supermarket, with the usual screaming kids and hassled-looking mothers. I was in a hurry—what else is new?—because I needed to get home and finish a report due that day, when a woman slipped ahead of me just as I joined the line. I found myself feeling impatient and resentful, time just seemed to stand still . . . and suddenly I realized what I was doing.

I stopped. I went inside myself, took a few deep breaths, and focused on my heart. An instant shift occurred, and I found a smile coming over my face. Instead of fighting my environment, I found myself at the center of it, and I relaxed. I waved at an adorable toddler, in a little jeans dress and matching hat, who had caught my eye moments earlier. Time did stand still now, but with an entirely different quality. I felt empathy with the checkout clerk, and gave her a friendly smile as I handed her my money. She smiled back.

We often feel helplessly pulled along by life. There are many moments each day when we can feel impatient, tense, and disconnected from both ourselves and others. But we are not helpless. We can turn these moments into opportunities to make contact, to acknowledge each other's humanity, to let warmth breed warmth. We do have a choice about how to perceive our world.

Optimism and a positive attitude go a long way in maintaining good health. Research shows that the higher one's optimism, the healthier one's immune system, and the more likely that good things will actually happen. Negative expectation, on the other hand, actually breeds negative experiences.

How do you incorporate these ideas and practices into your own life? You can begin by being grateful. No matter how bad things might appear, there is always someone who has worse problems. In fact, reaching out to such people may help you at least as much as it helps them! I have referred grieving widows and widowers, cancer survivors, and chronic fatigue patients to support groups of similar people, where they can use their experiences to help others.

One of the most basic skills is learning how to relax. Isn't it interesting that we have to learn this? Cats know how to relax automatically, as do babies. Their secret is being in the moment. Cats and babies don't think about paying the rent, getting to the dentist on time, or staying in relationships. They just are. How can we do this? I did it in the supermarket line. You can do it at a stoplight, in a bank line, or while waiting for your lunch date to arrive.

There are as many ways to relax as there are people. Go ahead and do something good for yourself. It does not have to be particularly expensive or time-consuming: a massage, a facial, a manicure. Take a quiet walk on the beach, or in a park, or in any special place where you can let go of your worries. Enjoy a beautiful sunset—I find nature to be the best soother of stress. Sometimes, even reminiscing about a pleasant experience in your past will cause your stress level to drop.

There are more structured forms of relaxation therapy. Yoga, meditation, biofeedback, self-hypnosis, tai chi, and other approaches can help you approach life with a greater sense of calm. Breathing exercises can also help (see "Breathing to Relax" on page 149). It takes only ten

to fifteen minutes per day to achieve a significant reduction in your depressive symptoms. If you want to
learn these techniques, look at the continuing education
catalogs from your area high school or college. Or keep
an eye on the announcements posted at your local library, community center, or house of worship. I find it
helps to use these techniques in a group: the group energy seems to prime the pump, making it easier to
reach a relaxed state. In addition, there are any number
of books and videos on these topics.

One last thing. Your feelings of depression or anxiety
just may be your mind's way of telling you to attend
to your spiritual needs, and for reasons that go beyond
simple stress reduction. For some people, the inspiration
gained from spirituality can be an essential part of the
healing process. Mind, body, and spirit are one, inseparable. Making an overt connection with the spirit will
provide healing for the mind and body.

HABITS TO AVOID

So far, I have covered the positive aspects of a depression-free lifestyle. Now it's time to look at several habits
you should avoid.

Smoking

Only someone living in a cave for the past twenty years
could be unaware of the health risks posed by tobacco
use. Heart disease, cancer, and stroke are the three big
killers in industrialized nations, and smoking is impli-
cated in all three. I grew up with a physician father
who had done cancer research, and who would preach
"no smoking" wherever he went, even though it was
not a popular subject at the time. None of us was ever
tempted to take up smoking.

Breathing to Relax

There are a number of relaxation techniques that focus on breath control. One involves focusing on the area below the navel and watching the breath as it goes in and out of your abdomen. Do this for five to ten minutes. This is a good sleep inducer.

Another breathing exercise is called the progressive relaxation response. Lie down and take several deep breaths. Then, breathe in slowly as you tense the muscles in your foot. Hold your breath, and the tension, for a count of twenty. (If you don't make it to twenty at the beginning, don't worry.) At twenty, slowly breathe out, releasing the muscles until they are totally relaxed. Repeat the process with your calf muscles, and work your way up, finishing with your facial muscles. Close with a few more deep breaths.

What you may not know is that smoking invites depression. It stimulates the secretion of adrenal hormones, including cortisol, which significantly reduces serotonin activity in the brain (see Chapter 3). In addition, the body uses much of its available supply of vitamin C to detoxify the byproducts of smoking, which can lead to a vitamin C deficiency. This can result in depression, apathy, weakness, and lowered immunity (see Chapter 8).

There is an ever-widening range of smoking cessation aids, from gums and patches to books and tapes. If you have a preexisting health problem, speak to your doctor before using any medicinal products.

Alcohol Consumption

Alcohol consumption can cause mood swings because it is tied to hypoglycemia (see page 136). Alcohol is a simple sugar, and is absorbed into the bloodstream directly from the stomach, without passing through the intestines. As a result, blood-sugar levels rise quickly, creating a type of sugar "high" that is part of alcohol's intoxicating effect. However, as we've seen, this excess sugar causes the body to produce more insulin, which causes blood-sugar levels to plummet. The reduction can trigger a desire for more alcohol or other simple sugars in order to restore blood-sugar levels. Unfortunately, such wide fluctuations in blood sugar ultimately contribute to a variety of mental and emotional problems, including depression.

There are nutrients that can help reduce the craving for alcohol, including the amino acid glutamine. Take 500 to 1,000 milligrams twice daily, or when a craving strikes. One man with a long history of alcoholism took my advice, and said that he was able to stop drinking entirely, while his twin brother continued to drink heavily. If you cannot control your drinking, seek help. Alcoholics Anonymous is only one of a number of organizations that can assist you in fighting your addiction.

Caffeine Consumption

Many people say they cannot get started in the morning without that first cup of coffee. Caffeine acts as a stimulant, enhancing short-term energy levels and increasing alertness. This sounds like an ideal solution to the problem of depression, except that depressed individuals tend to be more sensitive to caffeine than others. This frequently leads to a syndrome known as *caffeinism*, which can produce anxiety and panic disorders. Other symptoms of caffeinism include depression, irritability, nervousness, recurrent headaches, and heart palpitations. This problem can also affect people who drink many cans of caffeinated soft drinks each day.

My advice is to stop consuming caffeinated drinks altogether, since caffeine is so addictive. My coffee-craving patients are often hypoglycemic, and suffer from poor adrenal and/or thyroid function. The solution is improved diet, exercise, and specific supplements. As you reduce your body's dependence on caffeine, you will find that your overall energy level will rise.

In addition to knowing about St. John's wort and its synergistic supplements (discussed in Chapter 8), you know how to eat right, reduce your stress levels, and maintain good health habits. In the next chapter, I will leave you with some final thoughts on the natural approach to depression relief.

Conclusion

You now know how St. John's wort works, as well as when and how to use it for depression. We have discussed the research and clinical evidence of its effectiveness, and how it compares favorably with the synthetic antidepressants. We find in this herb an unusual combination of safety, effectiveness, broad range of positive effects, lack of side effects, and low cost.

St. John's wort has brought hope to millions of depressed people. There are those who have used antidepressants successfully, but prefer not to be dependent on a chemical substance for the rest of their lives, especially since we don't fully know the long-term effects of these drugs. Then, there is the majority of those on antidepressant medications who suffer from varying degrees of side effects, and who make calculated choices regarding their quality of life. They may accept the side effects as the price to pay for overcoming depression. Others will opt for stopping the medication, especially if the effects are severe enough, or if the trade-off is not worth it. Unfortunately for some, these effects have persisted despite their having stopped the drugs.

There are now new choices. Natural products provide a positive choice for many who would otherwise suffer from endless cycles of depression. As novel as these choices may seem, they are simply a return to traditional healing methods, ones our grandmothers used. (In fact, I discovered not long ago that my own maternal great-grandmother had been a respected herbalist and healer in her village in eastern Europe.) Those with mild to moderate depression can now be successfully treated with St. John's wort and other natural supplements without having to sacrifice quality of life or health to do so. For instance, in my own practice, I use natural hormone replacement therapy to treat my menopausal patients. There is no longer a need to choose between the risk of cancer with standard hormone replacement therapy on one hand, and menopausal symptoms, heart disease, and osteoporosis on the other. (For a list of natural medicine resources, see Appendix B.)

In addition, there are also many who simply cannot afford professional help, and who find that self-treatment with the herb is all they need. My professional preference is that individuals not self-diagnose and self-treat. However, there are economic realities that make professional help unavailable to many. In most developed countries, medical and mental health care is universally available. In the United States, however, mental health care, a stepchild of medicine, receives very poor support from medical insurers, and reform is sorely needed.

THE FUTURE OF HEALTH CARE

On a larger scale, St. John's wort's success has led to a renewed recognition and acceptance of herbal and natural medicine. It is bringing this entire field to the attention of the general population, which is looking beyond conventional medicine for solutions to health problems. Our dependence on technological medicine, including the use of pharmaceuticals, has not yielded increased freedom from disease. We are part of nature, and that is where we will find our own healing and balance. The molecular structure and energy fields of natural substances are much more compatible with our own biology than synthetics can ever be.

There is another important issue that must be raised. We are already exposed to so many chemical toxins in the environment that we don't need more in the form of drugs. Rather, we need to use herbal remedies in support of our bodies' efforts to process these toxins. For example, I will often treat those who are or have taken various drugs with herbs that support the liver, such as milk thistle. The liver detoxifies all the poisons to which we are exposed, and it needs all the help it can get.

This is an exciting time to be a physician, with many new possibilities for healing. I believe most doctors are motivated and curious to find the best, least harmful approaches to helping their patients. Many of my colleagues, previously skeptical of my interest and practice, now ask me for information on how to use a more natural approach. This field is growing so quickly that is difficult to keep up. Fortunately, patients who seek complementary care tend to be those most likely to take responsibility for their own healing, and least likely to expect the doctor to do or know it all. I would certainly never claim to have an all-encompassing knowledge about this ever-expanding field.

There are now many natural-medicine organizations that allow like-minded colleagues to share information, with their own journals and conferences. There are also more and more medical schools adding this field to their curriculum. There are still many skeptics, who always want more "proof." But even for them the evidence exists, and is constantly growing. On this note, I recommend that you take this book or others like it to your doctor to help inform him or her of the benefits of herbal medicine in general, and of St. John's wort in particular. Sharing this knowledge can help you, your doctor, and his or her other patients.

There is promising news in mainstream research possibilities. The National Institute of Mental Health (NIMH) is about to embark on a series of studies aimed at evaluating the efficacy and safety of a standardized hypericum extract in depression treatment. Perhaps we in this field can now work along with the government agencies, including the NIH and the FDA, to do research and to educate people about these effective, nontoxic treatments, which bring good health to all. Rising health costs are pointing the economic way toward these far less costly products.

PUTTING IT ALL TOGETHER

Whether we call the natural approach to medical care wholistic, alternative, orthomolecular, or complementary, it is the approach of the future. It is essential that we treat the whole person. St. John's wort is not simply a drug substitute, a natural "magic bullet" to replace the pharmaceutical ones. We cannot merely pop a pill, even an herbal one, for good health. No matter how natural and safe St. John's wort and other herbs may be, we still need to look for the root causes of disease, rather than just treating symptoms. For example, if a condition is psychologically based, it is important to explore issues and find psychological answers (see Chapter 2). If there is a metabolic or chemical imbalance anywhere in the body, it should be addressed as such (see Chapters 3 and 8).

Just as we cannot treat a symptom without looking at the entire body, we must also address the larger system in which we live. The increasing incidence of depression is directly proportional to the increasing levels of physical, chemical, and emotional stress to which we are exposed. This includes the toxic matter in our air, food, and water, the byproducts of runaway technology. The blatant disregard for the adverse effects of technology on the health of the planet will be remedied only by a return to nature, to the principles and conditions under which we have evolved and thrived.

Let us use St. John's wort as a bridge between conventional and alternative therapies, and continue to open up the vast realm of natural treatments. This expanded approach can lead us full circle to an increased appreciation of our natural resources. Sustaining what we have and renewing what we have destroyed is our only hope for the future—of humanity, of the planet, and of all living beings.

Appendix A

Suggested Readings

Chronic Fatigue Syndrome. Jay Goldstein. The Haworth Medical Press, Binghampton NY, 1993.

Dealing With Depression Naturally. Syd Baumel. Keats Publishing, New Canaan CT, 1995.

Eat Right for Your Type. Peter D'Adamo. Putnam, New York, 1996.

Embracing Your Inner Critic. Hal and Sidra Stone. HarperSanFrancisco, San Francisco, 1995.

EMDR. Francine Shapiro and Margot Silk Forrest. BasicBooks, New York, 1997.

Encyclopedia of Natural Medicine. Michael Murray and Joseph Pizzorno. Prima Publishing, Rocklin CA, 1994.

Five Steps to Selecting the Best Alternative Medicine. Mary and Michael Morton. New World Library, Novato CA, 1996.

40-30-30 Diet. Ann Louise Gittleman. Keats Publishing, New Canaan CT, 1997.

Healing Through Nutrition. Melvyn Werbach. Harper-Collins, New York, 1994.

Hormone Replacement Therapy, Yes or No. Betty Kamen. Nutrition Encounter, Inc., Novato CA, 1993.

Hypericum & Depression. Harold H. Bloomfield, Mikael Nordfors, and Peter McWilliams. Prelude Press, Los Angeles, 1996.

Hypothyroidism. Broda Barnes. Harper and Row, New York, 1976.

It's All in Your Head. Hal Huggins. Avery Publishing Group, Garden City Park NY, 1993.

Mastering the Zone. Barry Sears. Regan Books, New York, 1997.

Molecules of Emotion. Candace Pert. Scribner, New York, 1997.

Natural Alternatives to Prozac. Michael Murray. William Morrow and Co., New York, 1996.

The Natural Prozac Program. Jonathan Zuess. Three Rivers Press, New York, 1997.

The Nutrition Detective. Nan Fuchs. Tarcher, Los Angeles, 1985.

Omega-3 Oils. Donald Rudin and Clara Felix. Avery Publishing Group, Garden City Park NY, 1996.

Our Stolen Future. Theo Colborn, Dianne Dumanoski, and John Peterson Myers. Dutton, New York, 1996.

Prescription for Nutritional Healing. 2nd edition. James F. Balch and Phyllis A. Balch. Avery Publishing Group, Garden City Park NY, 1997.

The Real Vitamin and Mineral Book. 2nd edition. Shari Lieberman and Nancy Bruning. Avery Publishing Group,

Garden City Park NY, 1997.

Sacred Sorrows. John Nelson. Tarcher/Putnam, New York, 1996.

Say Good-bye to Illness. Devi Nambudripad. Delta Publishing, Buena Park CA, 1993.

The Serotonin Solution. Judith Wurtman. Fawcett Columbine, New York, 1997.

Solving the Puzzle of Chronic Fatigue Syndrome. Michael Rosenbaum and Murray Susser. Life Sciences Press, Tacoma WA, 1992.

Talking Back to Prozac. Peter Breggin. St. Martin's Paperback, New York, 1995.

Waking the Tiger Within. Peter Levine. North Atlantic Books, Berkeley CA, 1997.

The Way Up From Down. Priscilla Slagle. Random House, New York, 1987.

What Your Doctor May Not Tell You About Menopause. John Lee. Warner Books, New York, 1996.

Why We Get Sick. Randolph M. Nesse and George C. Williams. Random House, New York, 1995.

Why Zebras Don't Get Ulcers. Robert Sapolsky. W.H. Freeman and Co., New York, 1994.

Women's Bodies, Women's Wisdom. Christiane Northrup. Bantam, New York, 1994.

The Yeast Connection. William Crook. Professional Books, Jackson TN, 1983.

The Yeast Syndrome. John Parks Trowbridge. Bantam Books, New York, 1986.

Your Body Cries for Water. F. Batmanghelidj. Global Health Solutions, Falls Church VA, 1995.

Appendix B

Natural Medicine Resources

Alternative Medicine Resources

American College for Advancement in Medicine (ACAM)
P.O. Box 3427
Laguna Hills CA 96253
(714) 583-7666
(800) 532-3688

This is an organization of doctors and osteopaths who practice orthomolecular medicine, chelation therapy, and preventive medicine.

American Holistic Medical Association
4101 Lake Boone Trail
Suite 201
Raleigh NC 27607
(919) 787-5181

American Holistic Nurses' Association
4101 Lake Boone Trail
Suite 201
Raleigh NC 27607
(800) 278-AHNA
Fax: (919) 787-4916

American Medical Student Association
1902 Association Drive
Reston VA 22091
(703) 620-6600
Fax: (703) 620-5873

Canadian Holistic Medical Association
491 Eglinton Avenue West, #407
Toronto, Ont. M5N 1A8
(416) 485-3071

Center for Mind-Body Medicine
5225 Connecticut Avenue N.W.
Suite 414
Washington DC 20015
(202) 966-7338
Fax: (202) 966-2589

Holistic Health Directory
New Age Journal
42 Pleasant Street
Watertown MA 02172
(617) 926-0200

Office of Alternative Medicine
9000 Rockville Pike
Building 31, Room 5B-37
Mailstop 2182
Bethesda MD 20892
(301) 402-2466
Fax: (301) 402-4741

Acupuncture and Chinese Medicine

American Academy of Medical Acupuncture
5820 Wilshire Blvd
Suite 500
Los Angeles CA 90036
(213) 937-5514
Fax: (213) 937-0959
E-mail: KCKD71F@ prodigy.com

American Association of Acupuncture and Oriental Medicine
433 Front Street
Catasauqua PA 18032-2506

(610) 266-1433
Fax: (610) 264-2768

Biofeedback (including neurofeedback)

AAPB
10200 West 44th Avenue, Suite 304
Wheat Ridge CO 80033-2840
(303) 422-8436
Fax: (303) 422-8894
E-mail: aapb@resourcenter.com

Website: http://www.aapb.org/aapb.htm

Books and related material.

Flexyx, LLC
106 La Casa Via, Suite 110
Walnut Creek CA 94598
(510) 906-0422
Fax: (510) 906-0419
E-mail: lenochs@flexyx.com
Website: http://www.flexyx.com

Neurotherapy systems and clinical consulting.

Futurehealth, Inc.
3171 Rail Avenue
Trevose PA 19053
(215) 364-4445
Fax: (215) 364-4447
E-mail: infor@future health.org
Website: http://future-health.org

Chiropractic Medicine

American Chiropractic Association
1701 Clarendon Blvd
Arlington VA 22209
(703) 276-8800
(800) 986-4636
Fax: (703) 243-2593

International Chiropractors Association
1110 North Glebe Road
Suite 1000
Arlington VA 22201
(703) 528-5000

Clinical Nutrition

International and American Associations of Clinical Nutritionists (IAACN)
5200 Keller Springs Road, Suite 410
Dallas TX 75248
(972) 250-2829
Fax: (972) 250-0233

Compounding Pharmacies

Apothecure
13720 Midway
Dallas TX 75244
(800) 969-6601
Fax: (800) 687-5252
Website: http://www. apothecure.com

College Pharmacy
833 North Tejon Street
Colorado Springs CO 80903

(800) 888-9358
Fax: (800) 556-5893
Website: http://www. collegepharmacy.com

Medical Center Compounding Pharmacy
3675 South Rainbow Blvd, Suite 103
Las Vegas NV 89103
(800) 723-7455
Fax: (800) 238-8239
Website: http://www.mc-pharmacy.com

Women's International Pharmacy
13925 Meeker Blvd, Suite 13
Sun City West AZ 85375
(800) 279-5708
Fax: (800) 330-0268
Website: http://www. wipws.com

For one in your area, call International Acadamy of Compounding Pharmacists, (800) 927-4227

Environmental Medicine

American Academy of Environmental Medicine
10 East Randolph Street
New Hope PA
(215) 862-4544
Fax: (215) 862-4583

*Human Ecology Action
  League*
P.O. Box 29629
Atlanta GA 30359
(404) 248-1898

Herbal Medicine

American Botanical Council
P.O. Box 201660
Austin TX 78720
(512) 331-8868
Website: http://www.herbal
  gram.org

American Herbalists' Guild
P.O. Box 746555
Arvada CO 80006
(303) 423-8800
Fax: (303) 402-1564
E-mail: AHGoffice

Herb Research Foundation
1007 Pearl Street
Suite 200
Boulder CO 80302-9953
(303) 449-2265
(800) 748-2617
Fax: (303) 449-7849
Website: http://www.
  herbs.org

*Natural Product Research
  Consultants (NPRC)*
600 First Avenue, Suite 205
Seattle WA 98104
(206) 623-2520
E-mail:
  nprc@sttl.uswestnet.net
Website: http://www.nprc.
  com

*Publishes Quarterly Review of
  Natural Medicine and Clinical*

*Applications of Natural
  Medicine Monograph series—
  Depression, both for health care
  professionals; and Herbal
  Prescriptions for Better Health,
  for consumers.*

*Program for Collaborative
  Research in the
  Pharmaceutical Sciences*
M/C 877
College of Pharmacy—UIC
833 South Wood Street
Chicago IL 60612
(312) 996-2246

Herbal Suppliers—Mail Order

*Advanced Physcians
  Products*
831 State Street
Santa Barbara CA 93101
(800) 220-7687
Fax: (800) 438-6372
E-mail: app@silcom.com
website: htty://www.ap-
  products.com

Elixir Tonics and Teas
(888) 4-TONICS

Purity Products
1804 Plaza Avenue
New Hyde Park NY 11040
(800) 313-7873

Herbal Suppliers—Retail (through local sources)

Carlson Laboratories
22870 Iron Wedge Drive

Boca Raton FL 33433
(501) 395-9957

HerbPharm
Williams OR 97544
(800) 348-4372
Fax: (800) 545-7392
Tincture only.

Lichtwer Pharma U.S., Inc.
Pittsburgh PA 15220
(412) 928-9334

McZand Herbal
P.O. Box 5312
Santa Monica CA 90409
(800) 800-0405
Fax: (310) 822-1050

Nature's Plus
548 Broadhollow Road
Melville NY 11747
(800) 645-9500
Fax: (516) 249-2022

*Nutricology (Allergy
   Research Group)*
400 Preda Street
San Leandro CA 94577
(800) 545-9960
htty://www.nutricology.com

Planetary Formulations
P.O. Box 533
Soquel CA 95073
(800) 776-7701
Fax: (408) 438-7410

Homeopathic Medicine

*American Institute of
   Homeopathy*
1503 Glencoe
Denver CO 80220

(303) 898-5477

*Homeopathic Educational
   Services*
2124 Kittredge Street
Berkeley CA 94704
(510) 649-0294
Fax: (510) 649-1955
E-mail: mail@homeo
   pathic.com
Website: http://www.home-
   opathic.com

Light Therapy

*Environmental Health &
   Light Research Institute*
3923 Coconut Palm Drive
Suite 101
Tampa FL 33619
(800) 544-4878

Naturopathic Medicine

*American Association of
   Naturopathic Physicians*
2366 Eastlake Avenue E
Suite 322
Seattle WA 98102
(206) 323-7610

*Bastyr University of
   Natural Health Sciences*
14500 Juanita Drive
   Northeast
Bothell WA 98011
(425) 823-1300
Fax: (425) 823-6222
E-mail: admiss@bastyr.edu
Website: htty://www.
   bastyr.edu

The Canadian College of Naturopathic Medicine
2300 Yonge Street
18th Floor, Box 2431
Toronto, Ont. M4P IE4
(416) 486-8584

National College of Naturopathic Medicine
11231 S.E. Market Street
Portland OR 97216
(503) 255-4860
Fax: (503) 257-5929

Southwest College of Naturopathic Medicine and Health Sciences
6535 East Osborn Road
Suite 703
Scottsdale AZ 85251
(602) 990-7424
Fax: (602) 990-0337

Orthomolecular Medicine/Vitamin and Mineral Therapy

Linus Pauling Institute of Science and Medicine
440 Page Mill Road
Palo Alto CA 94306
(415) 327-4064

Price-Pottenger Nutrition Foundation
P.O. Box 2614
La Mesa CA 91943
(800) 366-3748

Orthomolecular Psychiatry

Well Mind Association of Greater Washington

11141 Georgia Avenue, #326
Wheaton MD 20902
(301) 949-8282

This organization provides a regular lecture series and referrals to alternative health practitioners.

Osteopathic Medicine

American Academy of Osteopathy
3500 DePauw Blvd
Suite 1080
Indianapolis IN 46268
(317) 879-1881

American Osteopathic Association
142 East Ontario Street
Chicago IL 60611
(312) 280-5800

Preventive Medicine

American Preventive Medical Association
459 Walker Road
Great Falls VA 22066
(800) 230-2762

Websites
The following alternative-health sites are in addition to those found in other listings, and include my own site:

http://www.doctorcass.com

http://www.arxc.com

http://www.healthy.net
(Health World Online)

Appendix C

Protocol for Switching a Patient from an Antidepressant to St. John's Wort

For mild depression, I use the following protocol. With SSRIs and tricyclics, I add 300 mg of St. John's wort while cutting the antidepressant dose in half. For example, if the patient is currently on 40 mg of Prozac a day, the dose is reduced to 20 mg a day. A 20-mg dose is reduced to 10 mg. Since Prozac has a long half-life, 20 mg every other day will have a similar effect as 10 mg daily, and will get around the necessity of supplying a new lower-dose prescription. Alternatively, the patient can empty the capsule, divide the contents, and take the divided doses on consecutive days.

I instruct the patient that if there is no apparent problem, after a week we will add another 300 mg of St. John's wort. A week later, a third capsule is added, bringing the daily dose to a full 900 mg. By the end of that week, the patient can discontinue the antidepressant. Generally this as a smooth process, with positive results. With more serious depression, I will leave the antidepressant at half strength for a month, in combination with the St. John's wort, then reevaluate, tapering off the medication as the full antidepressant effect of the herb is felt.

The program is different when changing from an MAOI to St. John's wort. Since we aren't certain of the mode of action of St. John's wort, and it appears to have some serotonin effect, it might cause a dangerous rise in blood pressure if mixed with an MAOI. To switch to St. John's wort in these cases would require a four-week washout period between stopping the drug and starting the herb.

Appendix D

The Regulatory Status of St. John's Wort in Various Countries

Australia   Included as an active ingredient in prod-
                   ucts listed in the Australian *Register of
                   Therapeutic Goods*.

Canada   Accepted traditional indications: seda-
                   tive, nervine, diuretic, and antispasmod-
                   ic in gastrointestinal disorders. Topical:
                   promotes wound-healing (vulnerary),
                   shrinks and soothes hemorrhoids (IPS,
                   1990). Currently under review.

Council of   Natural flavor source. Hypericin not to
Europe   exceed 0.1 mg/kg in finished food prod-
                   uct (Newall et al., 1996).

Czechoslovakia   Official in Pharmacopoeia (Reynolds,
                   1993).

ESCOP

Required to contain not less than 0.04% of naphthodianthrones of the hypericin group (total hypericin), calculated as hypericin. *Indications*: Mild to moderate depressive states (ICD-10 category F32.0, F32.1); somatoformic disturbances, including symptoms such as restlessness, anxiety, and irritability (ESCOP, 1996).

France

Approved for topical application as an emollient for urticaria, chaps, bruises, frostbite, insect bites, sunburns, and other minor burns, and for pain of the oral cavity or oropharynx (Bruneton, 1995).

Germany

German Drug Codex: Required to contain at least 0.04% of the hypericin group calculated as hypericin (DAC, 1986). *Indications*: Psychovegetative disturbances, depressive states, fear and/or nervous anxiety. *Oil preparations*: Dyspeptic conditions. *Approved external uses*: For the treatment and followup treatment of piercing and contused injuries, myalgia, first-degree burns (DAC, 1986). *Commission E*: Psychological disturbances, depression, anxiety, nervous unrest; oil for bruises due to trauma, myalgi, and first-degree burns (Blumenthal et al., 1997).

Poland

Official in Pharmacopoeia (Hobbs, 1989).

Romania

Official in Pharmacopoeia (Reynolds, 1993).

Russia

Official in Pharmacopoeia (Reynolds, 1993).

Switzerland
Required to contain a minimum of 0.08% total hypericin computed as hypericin (Pharmacopoeia Helvetica, 1996).

United Kingdom
Legal Category (Liscensed Products): GSL (for external use only; Newell et al., 1996). Occurs in British Herbal Pharmacopoeia. *Actions*: Sedative, astringent. *Topically*: Analgesic, antiseptic. *Indications*: Menopausal neurosis, excitability, neuralgia, fibrositis, sciatica (Bradley, 1983). *Topically*: Wounds.

United States
Regulated as a dietary supplement (PL:417). Approved as a natural flavoring in beverages, must be free of hypericin (Office of the Federal Registry, 1994).

With permission of Roy Upton, American Herbal Pharmacopoeia.

References

Chapter 2
Understanding Depression

Diagnostic and Statistical Manual of Mental Disorders IV. Washington DC: American Psychiatric Association, 1994, p. xxi.

Stone, Hal, and Stone, Sidra. *Embracing Your Inner Critic: Turning Self-Criticism Into a Creative Asset.* San Francisco: HarperSanFrancisco, 1995.

Chapter 3
The Mind, the Body, and Mental Health

Benkelfat, C. et al. Mood-lowering effect of tryptophan depletion. *Archives of General Psychiatry* 51:687–697, 1994.

Levine, Peter. *Waking the Tiger Within.* Berkeley CA: North Atlantic Books, 1997.

Pert, Candace. *Molecules of Emotion.* New York: Scribner, 1997.

Raleigh, M.J. et al. *Brain Research* 559:181–190, 1991. Cited in: Nesse, Randolph M., and Williams, George C. *Why We Get Sick: The New Science of Darwinian Medicine.* New York: Random House, 1995.

Sapolsky, Robert. *Why Zebras Don't Get Ulcers.* New York: W.H. Freeman and Co., 1994.

Shapiro, Francine, and Forrest, Margot Silk. *EMDR: The Breakthrough Therapy for Overcoming Anxiety, Stress, and Trauma.* New York: BasicBooks, 1997.

Thiele, B., Brink, I., Ploch, M. Modulation of cytokine expression by *Hypericum* extract *J. Geriatric Psychiatry Neurology*, 7(suppl 1):S60-62, 1994.

Chapter 4
St. John's Wort—The Versatile Herb

Barbagallo, C. and Chisari, G. Antimicrobial activity of three hypericum species. *Fitoterapia* 58:175–177, 1987.

Cooper, W. and James, J. An observational study of the safety and efficacy of hypericin in HIV+ subjects. *International Conference on AIDS* 6:369 (abstract 2063), 1990.

Cott and Misra 1997, in press. Cited in: *HerbalGram,* July 1997.

Evstifeeva, T.A., and Sibiriak, S.V. [The immunotropic properties of biologically active products obtained from Klamath weed (*Hypericum perforatum L.*).] *Eksperimentalnaia I Klinicheskaia Farmakologiia* 59(1):51–54, 1996.

Hobbs, Christopher. St. John's Wort: *Hypericum perforatum L. HerbalGram* 18/19:24–33, 1988/1989.

Lavie, D. Antiviral pharmaceutical compositions containing hypericin or pseudohypericin. European Patent Application No. 87111467.4, filed 8/8/87, European Patent Office, Publ. No. 0 256 A2, pp. 175–177, 1987.

Lavie, G., Mazur, Y. et al. Hypericin as an inactivator of infectious viruses in blood components. *Transfusion* 35(5):392–400, 1995.

Martinez, B.; Kasper, S; Ruhrmann, S.; and Möller, H.J. Hypericum in the treatment of seasonal affective disorders. *Journal of Geriatric Psychiatry and Neurology* 7(suppl 1):S29–S33, 1994.

Meruelo, D.; Lavie, G.; and Lavie, D. Therapeutic agents with dramatic antiretroviral activity and little toxicity at effective doses: Aromatic polycyclic diones hypericin and pseudohypericin. *Proceedings of the National Academy of Sciences USA* 85:5230–5234, 1988.

Muldner, V. and Zoller, M. Antidepressive wirkung eines auf den wirkstoffkomplex hypericin standardisierten hypericum-extrakes. *Arzneim Forsch* 34:918, 1984.

Perovic S and Muller WE. Pharmacological profile of hypericum extract. Effect on serotonin uptake by postsynaptic receptors. *Arzneimittelforschung* 45(11):1145–8, 1995.

Schulz, H. and Jobert, M. Effects of hypericum extract on sleep EEG in older volunteers. *Journal of Geriatric Psychiatry and Neurology* 7(suppl 1):S39–S43, 1994.

Smyshliaeva, A.V., and Kudriashov, IuB. [The modification of a radiation lesion with an aqueous extract of *Hypericum perforatum L.*] *Biologicheskie Nauki* 4:7–9, 1992.

Someya, H. Effect of constituent of *Hypericum erectum* on infection and multiplication of Epstein-Barr virus. *Journal of the Tokyo Medical College* 43:815–826, 1985.

Steinbeck-Klose, A. and Wernet, P. Succcessful long-term treatment over 40 months of HIV patients with intravenous hypericin. *International Conference on AIDS* 9(1): 470 (abstract PO-B26-2012), 1993.

Upton, Roy (ed). St. John's Wort: *Hypericum perforatum.* American Herbal Pharmacopoeia monograph, July 1997. Part of *HerbalGram*, July 1997.

Woelk, G.; Burkard, G.; and Gruenwald, J. Benefits and risks of the hypericum extract LI160: drug monitoring study with 3,250 patients. *Journal of Geriatric Psychiatry and Neurology* 7(suppl 1):S34–S38, 1994.

Notes for Inset on page 54

Berghöfer and Hölzl, 1989
Bystrov, 1975
Gurevich et al., 1971
Hölzl et al., 1989
Kitanov and Blinova, 1987
Lavie et al., 1995
Maisenbacher and Kovar, 1992
Nahrstedt and Butterweck, 1997
Olttmann et al., 1971
Sparenberg et al., 1993
Weber et al., 1994

Chapter 5
How to Use St. John's Wort

Bombardelli, E. and Morazzoni, P. *Hypericum perforatum. Fitoterapia* 66(1): 43–68, 1995.

Demisch, L.; Nispel, J.; Sielaff, T.; Gebhart, P.; Köhler, C.; Pflug, B. Influence of subchronic Hyperforat administration on melatonin production. *Pharmacopsychiatry* 1991.

Eckmann, F. Cerebral insufficiency treatment with ginkgo biloba extract: Time of onset of effect in a double-blind study with 60 inpatients. *Fortschr Med* 108:557–560, 1990.

Harrer, G. and Sommer, H. Treatment of mild/moderate depressions with hypericum. *Phytomedicine* 1:3–8, 1994.

Schubert et al. Depressive episode primarily unresponsive to therapy in elderly patients: Efficacy of ginkgo biloba in combination with antidepressants. *Geriatr Forsch* 3:45–53, 1993.

Sommer, H. and Harrer, G. Placebo-controlled double-blind study examining the effectiveness of an hypericum perparation in 105 mildly depressed patients. *Journal of Geriatric Psychiatry and Neurology* 7(suppl 1):S9–S11, 1994.

Staffeldt, B. et al. Pharmacokinetics of hypericin and pseudohypericin after oral intake of *Hypericum perforatum* extract LI160 in healthy volunteers. *Journal of Geriatric Psychiatry and Neurology* 7(suppl 1):S47–S53, 1994.

Suzuki, O.; Katsumata, Y.; and Oya, M. Inhibition of monoamine oxidase by hypericin. *Planta Medica* 43: 272–274, 1984.

Vorbach, E.U.; Hüber, W.D.; and Arnoldt, K.H. Effectiveness and tolerance of the hypericum extract LI160 in comparison with imipramine: randomized double-blind study with 135 outpatients. *Journal of Geriatric Psychiatry and Neurology* 7(suppl 1):S19–S23, 1994.

Witte, B. et al. Treatment of depressive symptoms with a high concentration hypericum preparation. A multicenter placebo-controlled double-blind study. *Fortschritte Der Medizin* 28:404–408, 1995.

Woelk, G.; Burkard, G.; and Gruenwald, J. Benefits and risks of the hypericum extract LI160: drug monitoring study with 3,250 patients. *Journal of Geriatric Psychiatry and Neurology* 7(suppl 1):S34–S38, 1994.

Chapter 6
Depression and St. John's Wort—Looking at the Proof

Martinez, B.; Kasper, S.; Ruhrmann, S.; and Möller, H.J. Hypericum in the treatment of seasonal affective disorders. *Journal of Geriatric Psychiatry and Neurology* 7(suppl 1):S29–S33, 1994.

Meruelo, D.; Lavie, G.; and Lavie, D. Therapeutic agents with dramatic antiretroviral activity and little toxicity at effective doses: Aromatic polycyclic diones hypericin and pseudohypericin. *Proceedings of the National Academy of Sciences USA* 85:5230–5234, 1988.

Hänsgren, K.; Vesper; and Ploch. Multicenter double-blind study examining the antidepressant effectiveness of the hypericum extract LI160. *Journal of Geriatric Psychiatry and Neurology* 7(suppl 1):S15–S18, 1994.

Harrer, G., and Sommer, H. Treatment of mild/moderate depressions with hypericum. *Phytomedicine* 1:3–8, 1994.

Harrer, G.; Hüber, W.D.; and Poduzweit, H. Effectiveness and tolerance of the hypericum extract LI160 compared to maprotiline: a multicenter double-blind study. *Journal of Geriatric Psychiatry and Neurology* 7(suppl 1):S24–S28, 1994.

Linde, K. et al. St. John's Wort for depression: an overview and meta-analysis of randomised clinical trials. *British Medical Journal* 313:253–258, 1996.

Suzuki, O.; Katsumata, Y.; and Oya, M. Inhibition of monoamine oxidase by hypericin. *Planta Medica* 43:272–274, 1984.

Vorbach, E.U.; Hüber, W.D.; and Arnoldt, K.H. Effectiveness and tolerance of the hypericum extract LI160 in comparison with imipramine: randomized double-blind study with 135 outpatients. *Journal of Geriatric Psychiatry and Neurology* 7(suppl 1):S19–S23, 1994.

Chapter 7
Prozac and Beyond—The Synthetic Antidepressants

Balon, R. et al. Sexual dysfunction during antidepressant treatment. *Journal of Clinical Psychiatry* 54:209–212, 1993.

Breggin, Peter. *Talking Back to Prozac.* New York: St. Martin's Paperback, 1995.

Henry, 1995. Cited in: Bloomfield, Harold H.; Nordfors, Mikael; and McWilliams, Peter. *Hypericum & Depression.* Los Angeles: Prelude Press, 1996.

Liebowitz, Michael R. *The Chemistry of Love.* New York: Little, Brown, 1983.

Chapter 8
Nutritional Approaches to Mental Health

Abou-Saleh, M.T. and Coppen, A. The biology of folate in depression: Implications for nutritional hypotheses of the psychoses. *Journal of Psychiatric Research* 20(2):91–101, 1986.

Ananth, J. and Yassa, R. Magnesium in mental illness. *Comprehensive Psychiatry* 20:475–482, September/October 1979.

Banderet, L.E. and Lieberman, H.R. Treatment with tyrosine, a neurotransmitter precursor, reduces environmental stress in humans. *Brain Research Bulletin* 22: 759–762, 1989.

Barnes, Broda. *Hypothyroidism.* New York: Harper and Row, 1976.

Beckmann, H. Phenylalanine in affective disorders. *Adv Biol Psychiatry* 10:137–147, 1983.

Birkmayer, W. et al. L-deprenyl plus L-phenylalanine in the treatment of depression. *Journal of Neural Transmission* 59:81–87, January 1984.

Braverman, Eric R., and Pfeiffer, Carl C. *The Healing Nutrients Within: Facts, Findings, and New Research on Amino Acids.* New Canaan CT: Keats Publishing, 1987.

Brush, M.G. and Perry, M. Pyridoxine and the premenstrual syndrome. *Lancet* 1399, 15 June 1985.

Carney, M.W.P. and Sheffield, B.F. Serum folic acid and B_{12} in 272 psychiatric inpatients. *Psychological Medicine* 8:139–144, 1978.

Carney, M.W.P. et al. Thiamine and pyridoxine lack in newly admitted psychiatric inpatients. *British Journal of Psychiatry* 135:239–254, 1979.

Carney, M.W.P. et al. Thiamine, riboflavin and pyridoxine deficiency in psychiatric inpatients. *British Journal of Psychiatry* 141:271–272, 1982.

Cox, I.M. et al. Red blood cell magnesium and chronic fatigue syndrome. *Lancet* 337:757–760, 30 March 1991.

Dubovsky, S.L. et al. Elevated platelet intracellular calcium concentration in bipolar depression. *Biol Psychiatry* 29:441–450, 1 March 1991.

Edwards, N. Mental disturbances related to metals. In Hall, Richard C.W. (ed): *Psychiatric Presentations of Medical*

Illness. Jamaica NY: Spectrum Publications, 1980, pp. 283–308.

Ellis, F.R. and Nasser, S. A pilot study of vitamin B_{12} in the treatment of tiredness. *British Journal of Nutrition* 30:277–283, 1973.

Fox, Arnold and Fox, Barry. *DLPA to End Chronic Pain and Depression.* New York: Pocket Books, 1985.

Gelenberg, A.J. et al. Neurotransmitter precursors for the treatment of depression. *Psychopharmacology Bulletin* 18(1): 7–18, 1982.

Gelenberg, A.J. et al. Tyrosine for depression: A double-blind trial. *Journal of Affective Diseases* 19:125–132, June 1990.

Kagan, B.L. Oral S-adenosylmethionine in depression: A randomized, double-blind, placebo-controlled trial. *American Journal of Psychiatry* 147:591–595, May 1990.

Lesser, Michael. *Nutrition and Vitamin Therapy.* New York: Grove Press, 1980.

Little, K.Y. et al. Altered zinc metabolism in mood disorder patients. *Biol Psychiatry* 26:646–648, October 1989.

McLoughlin, I.J. and Hodge, J.S. Zinc in depressive disorder. *Acta Psychiatria Scandinavica* 82:451–453, December 1990.

National Research Council. *Recommended Dietary Allowances.* 10th ed. Washington DC: National Academy Press, 1989.

Naylor, G.J. and Smith, A.H.W. Vanadium: A possible aetiological factor in manic depressive illness. *Psychological Medicine* 11:257–263, 1981.

Ohsawa, H. et al. An epidemiological study on hyponatremia in psychiatric patients in mental hospitals in Nara Prefecture. *Japanese Journal of Psychiatry and Neurology* 46:883–889, December 1992.

Ohta, T. et al. Daily activity and persistent sleep-wake schedule disorders. *Prog Neuro-Psychopharmacol Biol Psychiatry* 16:529–537, July 1992.

Osmond, H. and Hoffer, A. Massive niacin treatment in schizophrenia: Review of a nine-year study. *Lancet* I: 316–320, 1962.

Rosenbaum, J.F. et al. An open-label pilot study of oral S-adenosyl-L-methionine in major depression: Interim results. *Psychopharmacology Bulletin* 24(1):189–194, 1988.

Salmaggi, P. et al. Double-blind, placebo-controlled study of S-adenosyl-L-methionine in depressed postmenopausal women. *Psychother Psychosom* 59(1):34–40, 1993.

Thomson, J. et al. The treatment of depression in general practice: A comparison of L-tryptophan, amitriptyline, and a combination of L-tryptophan and amitriptyline with placebo. *Psychological Medicine* 12:741–751, November 1982.

van Praag, H.M. Management of depression with serotonin precursors. *Biol Psychiatry* 16(3):291–310, 1981.

Widmer, J. et al. Evolution of blood magnesium, sodium and potassium in depressed patients followed for three months. *Neuropsychobiology* 26(4):173–179, 1992.

Wynn, V. et al. Tryptophan, depression and steroidal contraception. *Journal of Steroid Biochemistry* 6:965–970, 1975.

Chapter 9
Living a Depression-Free Lifestyle

Calabrese, J.R. et al. Depression, immunocompetence, and prostaglandins of the E series. *Psychiatry Research* 17:41–47, 1985.

Erasmus, Udo. *Fats and Oils: The Complete Guide to Fats and Oils in Health and Nutrition.* Vancouver: alive, 1986.

Finnegan, John. *The Facts About Fats.* Malibu CA: Elysian Arts, 1993.

Lobstein, D.; Mosbacher, B.J.; and Ismail, A.H. Depression as a powerful discriminator between physically active and sedentary middle-aged men. *Journal of Psychosomatic Research* 27:69–76, 1983.

Rudin, D.O. The major psychoses and neuroses as omega-3 essential fatty acid deficiency syndrome: substrate pellagra. *Bio Psychiatry* 16:837–850, September 1981.

Appendix D
The Regulatory Status of St. John's Wort in Various Countries

Blumenthal, M.; Grünwald, J.; Hall, T.; Riggins, C.W.; and Rister, R.S. (eds); Klein, S. and Rister, R.S. (trans). *German Commission E Monographs: Therapeutic Monographs of Medicinal Plants for Human Use.* Austin TX: American Botanical Council, 1997 (at press).

Bradley, P. *British Herbal Pharacopoeia.* Bournemouth, Dorset, England: British Herbal Medicine Association, 1983.

Bruneton, J. *Pharmacognosy, Phytochemistry, Medicinal Plants.* Paris: Lavoisier Publishing, 1995.

DAC. *Deutscher Arzneimittel-Codex*. 3rd suppl 91 ed, 1986.

ESCOP. *Monograph: St. John's Wort*. European Scientific Co-operative for Phytomedicines. The Netherlands: Meppel, 1996.

Hobbs, C. St. John's Wort: *Hypericum perforatum L.* A review. *HerbalGram* 18/19:24–33, 1989.

IPS (Ingredient Policy Statement). *St. John's Wort*. Bureau of Nonprescription Drugs, Canada, 1990.

Newall, C.A.; Anderson, L.A.; and Phillipson, J.D. *Herbal Medicines: A Guide for Health-Care Professionals*. London: The Pharmaceutical Press, 1996.

Office of the Federal Registry, Publ. Code of Federal Regulations, Title 21. Washington DC: Food and Drug Administration, U.S. Government Printing Office, 1994.

Reynolds, J. *Martindale: The Extra Pharmacopoeia*. 30th ed. London: The Pharmaceutical Press, 1993.

Index